I0773871

MENOPAUSE BRAIN DIET COOKBOOK

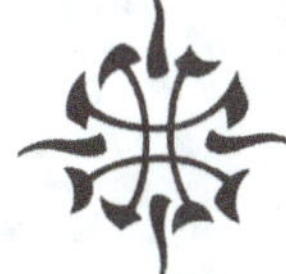

Nutritious and Delicious Recipes

Dr Megan L. Chupp

COPYRIGHTS

© [2024] by **Dr Megan L. Chupp**

All rights reserved. No part of this publication may be reproduced, distributed, or transmitted in any form or by any means, including photocopying, recording, or other electronic or mechanical methods, without the prior written permission of the publisher, except in the case of brief quotations embodied in critical reviews and certain other noncommercial uses permitted by copyright law.

Chapter 1:

Introduction:

Menopause is a natural phase in a woman's life that marks the end of her reproductive years. It typically occurs between the ages of 45 and 55, although the exact timing can vary from woman to woman. While menopause is commonly associated with physical changes such as hot flashes and hormonal fluctuations, it also affects cognitive function, leading to what is often referred to as "menopause brain."

Menopause brain refers to the cognitive changes and challenges that many women experience during the menopausal transition. It is characterized by symptoms such as memory lapses, difficulty concentrating, and mental fog. These cognitive changes can be frustrating and impact various aspects of a woman's life, including work, relationships, and overall well-being.

During menopause, a woman's body undergoes significant hormonal shifts. The primary hormones affected are estrogen and progesterone, which play a crucial role in brain function. Estrogen, in particular, influences neurotransmitters and promotes healthy blood flow to the brain. As estrogen levels decline during menopause, these changes can have an impact on cognitive abilities.

The exact mechanisms behind menopause brain are still not fully understood, but researchers believe that hormonal fluctuations and changes in brain structure and function contribute to these cognitive symptoms. It's important to note that not all women experience

6

menopause brain to the same extent, and the severity and duration of symptoms can vary.

In this book, we will explore the various aspects of menopause brain, providing insights, strategies, and practical advice for women navigating this transitional period. We will delve into the specific cognitive changes that occur during menopause, understand the factors that influence menopause brain, and discuss ways to manage and improve cognitive function. By gaining a deeper understanding of menopause brain, women can empower themselves to navigate this phase with confidence and maintain their cognitive well-being.

Menopause brings about a range of physical and hormonal changes, but it also has a significant impact on cognitive function. Many women notice changes in their memory, attention, and overall cognitive abilities during this transitional phase. Let's delve into these cognitive changes and understand how menopause can affect different aspects of cognitive function.

1. Memory:

Memory lapses and difficulties with recall are commonly reported by women going through menopause. These memory changes can manifest as forgetfulness, difficulty retrieving information, or experiencing "brain fog." The decline in estrogen levels is believed to play a role in these memory changes, as estrogen has a positive influence on memory processes. Furthermore, sleep disturbances and mood swings associated with menopause can also contribute to memory difficulties.

2. Attention and Concentration:

Maintaining focus and concentration can become more challenging during menopause. Women may find it harder to stay attentive, stay on task, or multitask effectively. This may be attributed to hormonal fluctuations affecting neurotransmitters in the brain, leading to reduced cognitive efficiency. Additionally, sleep disturbances, anxiety, and mood swings can further impact attention and concentration.

3. Processing Speed:

Menopause can also affect the speed at which information is processed by the brain. Women may notice a decline in their ability to quickly absorb and respond to new information. This slowed processing speed can be frustrating and may impact daily tasks that require swift mental processing, such as decision-making or problem-solving.

4. Executive Function:

Executive functions refer to higher-level cognitive processes involved in planning, organizing, problem-solving, and decision-making. Menopause can affect these executive functions, making it more challenging to manage complex tasks or juggle multiple responsibilities. Some women may experience difficulties in maintaining mental flexibility and adapting to new situations.

It's important to note that not all women will experience the same extent of cognitive changes during menopause. The severity and duration of symptoms can vary widely. Additionally, other factors such as age, overall health, lifestyle habits, and genetics can influence cognitive function during this phase.

Understanding memory lapses and brain fog

Memory lapses and brain fog are common cognitive symptoms experienced by many women during menopause. These can be frustrating and impact daily life, leading to difficulties in remembering names, finding words, or recalling recent events. Let's explore memory lapses and brain fog in more detail to understand their causes and potential strategies for managing them.

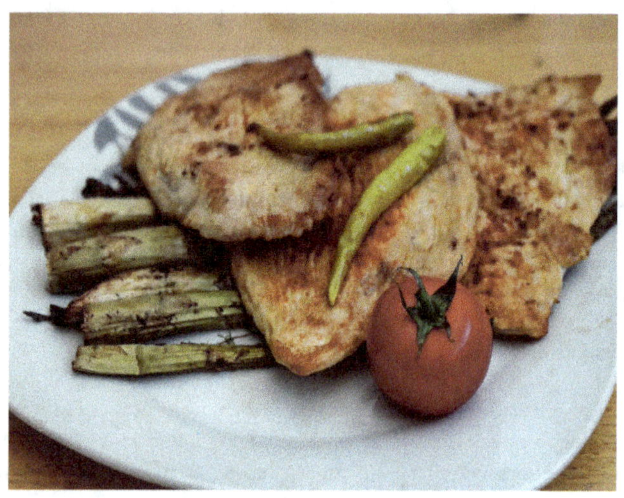

1. Memory Lapses:

Memory lapses during menopause often involve forgetfulness and occasional difficulty retrieving information. You may find yourself misplacing items more frequently or struggling to recall details of recent conversations. These memory changes can be attributed to several factors:

- Hormonal fluctuations: The decline in estrogen levels can affect the functioning of brain regions involved in memory processes. Estrogen plays a vital role in promoting healthy communication between brain cells and supporting memory formation and retrieval.

- Sleep disturbances: Menopause-related sleep problems, such as insomnia or night sweats, can disrupt the consolidation of memories during sleep. Inadequate sleep can impair memory consolidation and make it harder to retain new information.

- Stress and anxiety: Menopause is a time of significant hormonal and life changes, which can lead to increased stress and anxiety. High levels of stress hormones can interfere with memory and cognitive function.

2. Brain Fog:

Brain fog is a term used to describe a feeling of mental haziness or reduced mental clarity. It can make it challenging to concentrate, stay focused, and process information efficiently. Brain fog during menopause can be attributed to several factors:

- Hormonal changes: Fluctuating hormone levels, especially estrogen, can impact neurotransmitters in the brain that are essential for cognitive function. This can result in feelings of mental fatigue and foggy thinking.

- Sleep disturbances: Poor sleep quality or disrupted sleep patterns can contribute to brain fog. When you don't get enough restorative sleep, it can affect cognitive performance and contribute to mental cloudiness.

- Mood changes: Mood swings, anxiety, and depression are common during menopause. These emotional fluctuations can affect cognitive function and contribute to brain fog.

Managing Memory Lapses and Brain Fog:

While memory lapses and brain fog can be challenging, there are strategies you can employ to manage and improve cognitive function during menopause:

- Stay mentally active: Engaging in mentally stimulating activities, such as puzzles, reading, or learning new skills, can help keep your brain sharp and enhance memory function.

- Maintain a healthy lifestyle: Regular exercise, a balanced diet, and adequate sleep are crucial for optimal cognitive function. Exercise improves blood flow to the brain and promotes the release of endorphins, which can enhance mood and cognition.

- Practice stress management: Incorporate stress-reducing techniques into your daily routine, such as meditation, deep breathing exercises, or engaging in hobbies that bring you joy and relaxation.

- Seek social support: Connecting with others and sharing experiences can provide emotional support during this transitional phase. Surround yourself with a supportive network of friends and family.

- Consider hormone therapy: Hormone replacement therapy (HRT) may be an option for managing menopause symptoms, including cognitive changes. Consult with your healthcare provider to determine if it's suitable for you.

By understanding the causes of memory lapses and brain fog during menopause and implementing these strategies, you can navigate through these cognitive challenges with greater ease and maintain mental clarity and well-being.

Experiencing cognitive changes during menopause can be challenging, but there are various strategies you can employ to manage and improve your cognitive function. By incorporating these strategies into your daily routine, you can enhance your mental clarity and overall cognitive well-being. Let's explore some effective strategies for managing cognitive changes during menopause:

1. Maintain a Healthy Lifestyle:

- Regular exercise: Engaging in physical activity promotes healthy blood flow to the brain, enhances mood, and improves cognitive function. Aim for at least 30 minutes of moderate-intensity exercise, such as brisk walking, swimming, or cycling, most days of the week.

- Balanced diet: Nourishing your body with a well-balanced diet rich in fruits, vegetables, whole grains, lean proteins, and healthy fats provides essential nutrients for brain health. Include foods high in antioxidants, such as berries and leafy greens, which can protect brain cells from oxidative stress.

- Quality sleep: Prioritize good sleep hygiene by establishing a consistent sleep schedule, creating a relaxing bedtime routine, and ensuring a comfortable sleep environment. Quality sleep is crucial for memory consolidation and optimal cognitive function.

- Stress management: Chronic stress can negatively impact cognitive function. Explore stress-reducing techniques that work for you, such as mindfulness meditation, deep breathing exercises, yoga, or engaging in hobbies and activities that bring you joy and relaxation.

2. Mental Stimulation:

- Engage in mentally challenging activities: Regularly engage in activities that stimulate your brain, such as puzzles, crosswords, reading, learning new skills, or playing strategy games. These activities help keep your mind active and promote cognitive flexibility.

- Lifelong learning: Pursue new interests and continue learning throughout your life. Take up a new hobby, enroll in classes or workshops, or explore online courses. Lifelong learning not only keeps your brain engaged but also fosters personal growth and fulfillment.

- Cognitive exercises: Specific cognitive exercises, such as memory games, attention-training tasks, and brain-training apps, can help sharpen cognitive skills and improve memory, attention, and processing speed.

3. Organization and Time Management:

- Use calendars and reminders: Utilize calendars, planners, or smartphone apps to keep track of appointments, tasks, and important dates. Set reminders and alarms to help you stay organized and prompt your memory.

- Break tasks into smaller steps: When faced with complex tasks or projects, break them down into smaller, manageable steps. This approach can help reduce overwhelm and improve focus and productivity.

- Prioritize and delegate: Recognize your priorities and delegate tasks when necessary. Streamlining your to-do list and focusing on essential activities can help reduce cognitive load and enhance efficiency.

4. Support and Self-Care:

- Seek social support: Surround yourself with a supportive network of family and friends. Sharing experiences, receiving emotional support, and engaging in social activities can positively impact your mood and cognitive well-being.

- Self-care practices: Prioritize self-care to promote overall well-being. Engage in activities that bring you joy, relaxation, and fulfillment. This may include hobbies, creative outlets, spending time in nature, practicing self-compassion, or seeking professional counseling if needed.

- Stay positive and patient: Be patient with yourself during this transitional phase. Practice positive self-talk, celebrate small victories, and maintain a growth mindset. Remember that cognitive changes during menopause are often temporary and manageable.

It's essential to consult with your healthcare provider if you have concerns about cognitive changes during menopause. They can provide personalized guidance, recommend appropriate interventions, and address any underlying medical conditions that may contribute to cognitive symptoms.

Chapter 2:

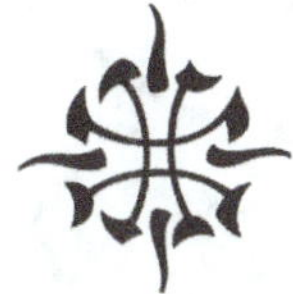

BOOSTING MEMORY AND COGNITIVE FUNCTION

Blueberry Brain Smoothie:

Ingredients:

- 1 cup blueberries (fresh or frozen)

- 1 ripe banana

- 1 cup spinach

- 1 tablespoon chia seeds

- 1 cup almond milk (or your preferred plant-based milk)

- 1 tablespoon honey or maple syrup (optional for added sweetness)

Preparation:

1. Place all the ingredients in a blender.

2. Blend until smooth and creamy.

3. If desired, adjust the sweetness by adding honey or maple syrup.

4. Pour into a glass and enjoy!

Prep time: Approximately 5 minutes

Ingredients:

- 1 salmon fillet

- Salt and pepper to taste

- 4 cups mixed salad greens

- 1 ripe avocado, sliced

- 1/2 cup cherry tomatoes, halved

- 1/4 red onion, thinly sliced

- 2 tablespoons lemon juice

- 1 tablespoon extra-virgin olive oil

Preparation:

1. Preheat the oven to 400°F (200°C).

2. Season the salmon fillet with salt and pepper.

3. Place the salmon on a baking sheet lined with parchment paper and bake for 12-15 minutes or until cooked through.

4. In a large bowl, combine the salad greens, avocado slices, cherry tomatoes, and red onion.

5. In a small bowl, whisk together the lemon juice and olive oil to make the dressing.

6. Flake the cooked salmon and add it to the salad.

7. Drizzle the dressing over the salad and gently toss to combine.

8. Serve the salad immediately.

Prep time: Approximately 20 minutes

Ingredients:

- 2 boneless, skinless chicken breasts

- Salt and pepper to taste

- 2 cups fresh spinach leaves

- 1/4 cup chopped walnuts

- 2 tablespoons grated Parmesan cheese

- 1 tablespoon olive oil

Preparation:

1. Preheat the oven to 375°F (190°C).

2. Butterfly the chicken breasts by cutting horizontally through the middle, but not all the way through.

3. Season the inside of each chicken breast with salt and pepper.

4. In a small bowl, combine the spinach, walnuts, and Parmesan cheese.

5. Stuff each chicken breast with the spinach mixture and secure with toothpicks if needed.

6. Heat the olive oil in an oven-safe skillet over medium-high heat.

7. Sear the stuffed chicken breasts for 2-3 minutes on each side until lightly browned.

8. Transfer the skillet to the preheated oven and bake for 15-20 minutes or until the chicken is cooked through.

9. Remove from the oven and let the chicken rest for a few minutes before serving.

Prep time: Approximately 30 minutes

Quinoa and Vegetable Stir-Fry:

Ingredients:

- 1 cup quinoa

- 2 cups vegetable broth or water

- 1 tablespoon olive oil

- 1 onion, diced

- 2 cloves garlic, minced

- 1 bell pepper, sliced

- 1 zucchini, sliced

- 1 cup broccoli florets

- 1 cup snap peas

- 2 tablespoons low-sodium soy sauce (or tamari for a gluten-free option)

- 1 tablespoon sesame oil (optional)

- Salt and pepper to taste

- Fresh cilantro or green onions for garnish

Preparation:

1. Rinse the quinoa thoroughly under cold water.

2. In a saucepan, bring the vegetable broth or water to a boil and add the quinoa. Reduce heat, cover, and simmer for about 15-20 minutes or until the quinoa is cooked and the liquid is absorbed.

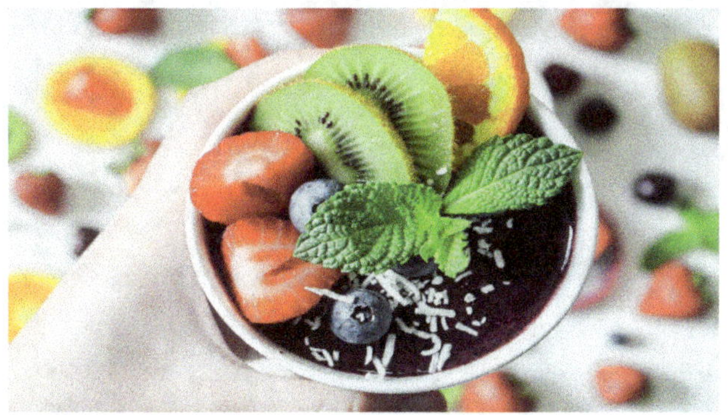

3. In a large skillet or wok, heat the olive oil over medium-high heat.

4. Add the diced onion and minced garlic, and sauté until fragrant and the onion becomes translucent.

5. Add the bell pepper, zucchini, broccoli, and snap peas to the skillet. Stir-fry for about 5-7 minutes, or until the vegetables are tender-crisp.

6. Stir in the cooked quinoa, soy sauce, and sesame oil (if using). Season with salt and pepper to taste.

7. Continue to cook for a few more minutes, stirring to combine all the flavors.

8. Garnish with fresh cilantro or green onions before serving.

Prep time: Approximately 30 minutes

Turmeric Roasted Cauliflower:

Ingredients:

- 1 large cauliflower head, cut into florets

- 2 tablespoons olive oil

- 1 teaspoon turmeric powder

- 1/2 teaspoon cumin powder

- 1/2 teaspooncoriander powder

- 1/2 teaspoon paprika

- Salt and pepper to taste

- Fresh parsley or cilantro for garnish

Preparation:

1. Preheat the oven to 425°F (220°C).

2. In a large bowl, combine the cauliflower florets, olive oil, turmeric powder, cumin powder, coriander powder, paprika, salt, and pepper. Toss until the cauliflower is evenly coated.

3. Spread the cauliflower in a single layer on a baking sheet lined with parchment paper.

4. Roast in the preheated oven for 25-30 minutes, or until the cauliflower is tender and golden brown, stirring once or twice during cooking.

5. Remove from the oven and garnish with fresh parsley or cilantro before serving.

Prep time: Approximately 35 minutes

Ingredients:

- 1/4 cup chia seeds

- 1 cup almond milk (or your preferred plant-based milk)

- 1 tablespoon honey or maple syrup

- 1/2 teaspoon vanilla extract

- Fresh berries (such as strawberries, blueberries, or raspberries) for topping

Preparation:

1. In a bowl, combine the chia seeds, almond milk, honey or maple syrup, and vanilla extract.

2. Stir well to ensure the chia seeds are evenly distributed.

3. Let the mixture sit for about 5 minutes, then stir again to prevent clumping.

4. Cover the bowl and refrigerate for at least 2 hours or overnight, allowing the chia seeds to absorb the liquid and thicken.

5. Once the pudding has reached the desired consistency, give it a final stir.

6. Serve the chia seed pudding in individual bowls or jars and top with fresh berries.

7. Enjoy chilled!

Prep time: Approximately 5 minutes (+ chilling time)

Ingredients:

- 2 cups broccoli florets

- 1 tablespoon olive oil

- 1 small onion, chopped

- 2 cloves garlic, minced

- 3 cups vegetable broth

- 1/4 cup almond butter

- Salt and pepper to taste

- Sliced almonds for garnish

Preparation:

1. In a large pot, heat the olive oil over medium heat.

2. Add the chopped onion and minced garlic, and sauté until the onion becomes translucent.

3. Add the broccoli florets to the pot and cook for a few minutes until slightly softened.

4. Pour in the vegetable broth and bring the mixture to a boil. Reduce the heat and simmer for about 10 minutes, or until the broccoli is tender.

5. Remove the pot from heat and let it cool slightly.

6. Using an immersion blender or a regular blender, puree the soup until smooth.

7. Return the soup to the pot and stir in the almond butter until well combined.

8. Season with salt and pepper to taste.

9. Reheat the soup if necessary before serving.

10. Garnish each serving with sliced almonds.

Prep time: Approximately 25 minutes

Ingredients:

- 2 medium sweet potatoes, peeled and diced

- 1 tablespoon olive oil

- 1 small onion, chopped

- 2 cloves garlic, minced

- 2 cups kale leaves, chopped

- 1 teaspoon smoked paprika

- 1/2 teaspoon cumin

- Salt and pepper to taste

- Fresh parsley for garnish

Preparation:

1. In a large skillet, heat the olive oil over medium heat.

2. Add the chopped onion and minced garlic, and sauté until the onion becomes translucent.

3. Add the diced sweet potatoes to the skillet and cook for about 10 minutes, stirring occasionally, until they are slightly tender.

4. Stir in the chopped kale leaves, smoked paprika, cumin, salt, and pepper.

5. Continue cooking for another 5-7 minutes, or until the sweet potatoes are cooked through and the kale is wilted.

6. Remove from heat and garnish with fresh parsley before serving.

Prep time: Approximately 25 minutes

Ingredients:

- 8 ounces dark chocolate (70% cocoa or higher), chopped

- 1/4 cup mixed nuts (such as almonds, walnuts, or cashews), chopped

- 2 tablespoons mixed seeds (such as pumpkin seeds or sunflower seeds)

- Dried cranberries or other dried fruits (optional)

- Pinch of sea salt (optional)

Preparation:

1. Line a baking sheet with parchment paper.

2. In a heatproof bowl, melt the dark chocolate either in the microwave or using a double boiler, stirring until smooth.

3. Pour the melted chocolate onto the prepared baking sheet and spread it out into an even layer.

4. Sprinkle the chopped nuts, seeds, and dried cranberries (if using) evenly over the chocolate.

5. If desired, sprinkle a pinch of sea salt over the top for a savory-sweet flavor.

6. Place the baking sheet in the refrigerator for about 30 minutes, or until the chocolate has fully hardened.

7. Once hardened, break the chocolate bark into smaller pieces.

8. Store in an airtight container in a cool place or the refrigerator until ready to serve.

Prep time: Approximately 10 minutes (+ chilling time)

Ingredients:

- 2 salmon fillets

- 2 tablespoons olive oil

- 3 cloves garlic, minced

- 1 tablespoon chopped fresh herbs (such as dill, parsley, or thyme)

- Juice of 1/2 lemon

- Salt and pepper to taste

- Lemon slices for garnishPreparation:

1. Preheat the oven to 400°F (200°C).

2. Place the salmon fillets on a baking sheet lined with parchment paper.

3. In a small bowl, combine the olive oil, minced garlic, chopped fresh herbs, lemon juice, salt, and pepper. Stir well to make a marinade.

4. Brush the marinade over the salmon fillets, ensuring they are evenly coated.

5. Place a few lemon slices on top of each fillet for added flavor.

6. Bake in the preheated oven for about 12-15 minutes, or until the salmon is cooked to your desired doneness.

7. Remove from the oven and let the salmon rest for a couple of minutes before serving.

8. Serve the roasted salmon with your choice of sides, such as steamed vegetables or a salad.

Prep time: Approximately 20 minutes

Ingredients:

- 4 cups baby spinach leaves

- 1 cup mixed berries (such as strawberries, blueberries, and raspberries)

- 1/4 cup crumbled goat cheese

- 1/4 cup sliced almonds

- Balsamic vinaigrette (homemade or store-bought)

Preparation:

1. In a large salad bowl, combine the baby spinach leaves, mixed berries, crumbled goat cheese, and sliced almonds.

2. Drizzle the desired amount of balsamic vinaigrette over the salad.

3. Toss gently to coat all the ingredients with the dressing.

4. Serve immediately as a refreshing and healthy salad.

Prep time: Approximately 10 minutes

Ingredients:

- 8 ounces pasta of your choice

- 1 pound shrimp, peeled and deveined

- 3 tablespoons olive oil

- 4 cloves garlic, minced

- Zest and juice of 1 lemon

- 1/4 teaspoon red pepper flakes (optional)

- Salt and pepper to taste

- Chopped fresh parsley for garnish

Preparation:

1. Cook the pasta according to the package instructions until al dente. Drain and set aside.

2. In a large skillet, heat the olive oil over medium heat.

3. Add the minced garlic and sauté for about 1 minute until fragrant.

4. Add the shrimp to the skillet and cook for 2-3 minutes per side, or until they turn pink and opaque.

5. Stir in the lemon zest, lemon juice, red pepper flakes (if using), salt, and pepper. Cook for an additional minute to allow the flavors to meld.

6. Add the cooked pasta to the skillet and toss to coat the pasta with the lemon garlic sauce.

7. Remove from heat and garnish with chopped fresh parsley.

8. Serve the lemon garlic shrimp pasta immediately.

Prep time: Approximately 20 minutes

Ingredients:

- 4 medium beets, peeled and cubed

- 2 tablespoons olive oil

- Salt and pepper to taste

- 4 cups mixed salad greens

- 1/2 cup crumbled goat cheese

- 1/4 cup walnuts, chopped

- Balsamic vinaigrette (homemade or store-bought)

Preparation:

1. Preheat the oven to 400°F (200°C).

2. In a large bowl, toss the cubed beets with olive oil, salt, and pepper until well coated.

3. Spread the beets in a single layer on a baking sheet lined with parchment paper.

4. Roast in the preheated oven for about 25-30 minutes, or until the beets are tender when pierced with a fork.

5. Remove the beets from the oven and let them cool slightly.

6. In a salad bowl, combine the mixed salad greens, roasted beets, crumbled goat cheese, and chopped walnuts.

7. Drizzle balsamic vinaigrette over the salad and toss gently to combine.

8. Serve the roasted beet and goat cheese salad as a delightful and colorful side dish or main course.

Prep time: Approximately 40 minutes

Pumpkin and Lentil Curry:

Ingredients:

- 1 tablespoon olive oil

- 1 onion, chopped

- 3 cloves garlic, minced

- 1 tablespoon grated ginger

- 2 tablespoons curry powder

- 1 teaspoon ground cumin

- 1/2 teaspoon ground turmeric

- 1/4 teaspoon cayenne pepper (optional, adjust to taste)

- 1 cup red lentils

- 2 cups pumpkin or butternut squash, peeled and cubed

- 1 can (14 ounces) coconut milk

- 2 cups vegetable broth

- Salt and pepper to taste

- Fresh cilantro for garnish

- Cooked rice or naan bread for serving

Preparation:

1. In a large pot, heat the olive oil over medium heat.

2. Add the chopped onion, minced garlic, and grated ginger. Sauté until the onion becomes translucent.

3. Stir in the curry powder, ground cumin, ground turmeric, and cayenne pepper (if using). Cook for another minute to toast the spices and release their flavors.

4. Add the red lentils, cubed pumpkin or butternut squash, coconut milk, and vegetable broth to the pot. Stir well to combine.

5. Bring the mixture to a boil, then reduce the heat and simmer, covered, for about 20-25 minutes, or until the lentils and pumpkin/squash are tender.

6. Season with salt and pepper to taste.

7. Serve the pumpkin and lentil curry over cooked rice or with naan bread.

8. Garnish with fresh cilantro before serving.

Prep time: Approximately 40 minutes

Greek Yogurt Parfait with Granola:

Ingredients:

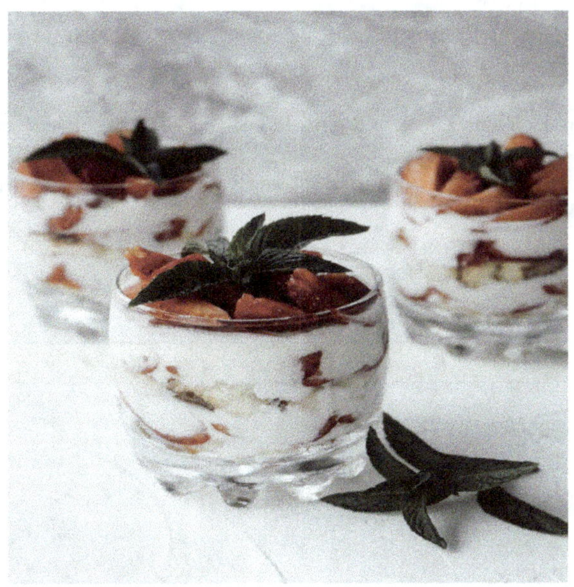

- 1 cup Greek yogurt

- 1 tablespoon honey or maple syrup

- 1/2 teaspoon vanilla extract

- 1 cup mixed berries (such as strawberries, blueberries, and raspberries)

- 1/2 cup granola (homemade or store-bought)

Preparation:

1. In a bowl, combine the Greek yogurt, honey or maple syrup, and vanilla extract. Stir well to incorporate the sweetener and flavor.

2. In a glass or a serving dish, layer half of the Greek yogurt mixture.

3. Add a layer of mixed berries on top of the yogurt.

4. Sprinkle a layer of granola over the berries.

5. Repeat the layers with the remaining Greek yogurt mixture, berries, and granola.

6. Finish off with a final layer of berries and a sprinkle of granola on top.

7. Serve the Greek yogurt parfait immediately as a delicious and nutritious breakfast or snack.

Prep time: Approximately 5 minutes

Baked Cod with Lemon and Dill:

Ingredients:

- 4 cod fillets

- 2 tablespoons olive oil

- Juice of 1 lemon

- Zest of 1 lemon

- 2 cloves garlic, minced

- 2 tablespoons fresh dill, chopped

- Salt and pepper to taste

- Lemon wedges for serving

Preparation:

1. Preheat the oven to 400°F (200°C) and lightly grease a baking dish.

2. Place the cod fillets in the prepared baking dish.

3. In a small bowl, whisk together the olive oil, lemon juice, lemon zest, minced garlic, chopped dill, salt, and pepper.

4. Pour the mixture over the cod fillets, ensuring they are evenly coated.

5. Bake in the preheated oven for about 12-15 minutes, or until the fish flakes easily with a fork.

6. Serve the baked cod with lemon and dill with lemon wedges on the side.

Prep time: Approximately 20 minutes

Ingredients:

- 1 cup dates, pitted

- 1 cup unsweetened shredded coconut

- Zest of 1 lime

- Juice of 1 lime

- 1/4 cup almond flour

- 2 tablespoons chia seeds

- 1 tablespoon honey or maple syrup (optional, for added sweetness)

- Extra shredded coconut for rolling (optional)

Preparation:

1. Place the pitted dates, shredded coconut, lime zest, lime juice, almond flour, chia seeds, and honey or maple syrup (if using) in a food processor.

2. Process the ingredients until they form a sticky mixture that holds together when pressed between your fingers.

3. Scoop out small portions of the mixture and roll them into bite-sized balls.

4. If desired, roll the energy balls in additional shredded coconut for an extra coating.

5. Place the energy balls on a baking sheet lined with parchment paper and refrigerate for at least 30 minutes to set.

6. Once set, transfer the coconut lime energy balls to an airtight container and store them in the refrigerator for up to one week.

7. Enjoy these delicious and energizing snacks whenever you need a quick boost!

Prep time: Approximately 15 minutes

Ingredients:

- 4 bell peppers (any color)

- 1 cup cooked quinoa

- 1 cup black beans, rinsed and drained

- 1 cup corn kernels (fresh or frozen)

- 1/2 cup diced tomatoes

- 1/2 cup shredded cheddar cheese

- 1/4 cup chopped fresh cilantro

- 1 teaspoon ground cumin

- 1/2 teaspoon chili powder

- Salt and pepper to taste

Preparation:

1. Preheat the oven to 375°F (190°C) and lightly grease a baking dish.

2. Cut the tops off the bell peppers and remove the seeds and membranes from the inside.

3. In a large bowl, combine the cooked quinoa, black beans, corn kernels, diced tomatoes, shredded cheddar cheese, chopped cilantro, ground cumin, chili powder, salt, and pepper. Mix well.

4. Spoon the quinoa and black bean mixture into the hollowed-out bell peppers, packing it tightly.

5. Place the stuffed bell peppers in the greased baking dish.

6. Cover the baking dish with foil and bake in the preheated oven for 25 minutes.

7. Remove the foil and bake for an additional 10-15 minutes, or until the bell peppers are tender and the filling is heated through.

8. Serve the quinoa and black bean stuffed bell peppers as a tasty and nutritious main course.

Prep time: Approximately 40 minutes

Roasted Brussels Sprouts with Bacon:

Ingredients:

- 1 pound Brussels sprouts, trimmed and halved

- 4 slices bacon, cooked and crumbled

- 2 tablespoons olive oil

- Salt and pepper to taste

Preparation:

1. Preheat the oven to 400°F (200°C) and line a baking sheet with parchment paper.

2. In a large bowl, toss the Brussels sprouts with olive oil, salt, and pepper until well coated.

3. Spread the Brussels sprouts in a single layer on the prepared baking sheet.

4. Roast in the preheated oven for about 20-25 minutes, or until the sprouts are tender and lightly browned, stirring once or twice during cooking.

5. Remove the roasted Brussels sprouts from the oven and transfer them to a serving dish.

6. Sprinkle the crumbled bacon over the top.

7. Serve the roasted Brussels sprouts with bacon as a flavorful side dish.

Prep time: Approximately 30 minutes

Mango and Avocado Salsa:

Ingredients:

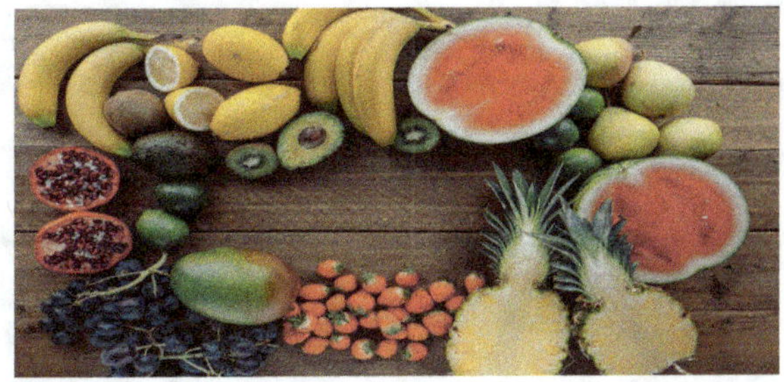

- 1 ripe mango, peeled, pitted, and diced- 1 ripe avocado, peeled, pitted, and diced

- 1/2 red onion, finely chopped

- 1 jalapeño pepper, seeded and finely chopped

- Juice of 1 lime

- 2 tablespoons chopped fresh cilantro

- Salt and pepper to taste

Preparation:

1. In a bowl, combine the diced mango, diced avocado, finely chopped red onion, finely chopped jalapeño pepper, lime juice, chopped cilantro, salt, and pepper.

2. Gently toss the ingredients together until well mixed.

3. Taste and adjust the seasoning if needed.

4. Allow the salsa to sit for about 10-15 minutes to allow the flavors to meld together.

5. Serve the mango and avocado salsa as a refreshing and vibrant topping for grilled meats, fish, tacos, or as a dip with tortilla chips.

Prep time: Approximately 15 minutes

Enjoy these delicious and diverse recipes! Feel free to modify them according to your taste preferences and dietary needs.

Chapter 3:

Mᴏᴏᴅ-Bᴏᴏsᴛɪɴɢ Rᴇᴄɪᴘᴇs

Chocolate Banana Smoothie:

Ingredients:

- 1 ripe banana

- 1 cup milk (dairy or plant-based)

- 1 tablespoon cocoa powder

- 1 tablespoon honey or maple syrup (optional, for added sweetness)

- 1/2 teaspoon vanilla extract

- Ice cubes (optional)

Preparation:

1. Peel the ripe banana and break it into chunks.

2. Place the banana chunks, milk, cocoa powder, honey or maple syrup (if using), and vanilla extract in a blender.

3. Blend the ingredients until smooth and creamy.

4. If desired, add a few ice cubes to the blender and blend again until the smoothie is chilled and frothy.

5. Pour the chocolate banana smoothie into a glass and enjoy it as a delicious and satisfying treat.

Prep time: Approximately 5 minutes

Caprese Salad Skewers:

Ingredients:

- Cherry tomatoes

- Fresh mozzarella balls (bocconcini)

- Fresh basil leaves

- Balsamic glaze (store-bought or homemade)

- Skewers or toothpicks

Preparation:

1. Rinse the cherry tomatoes and pat them dry.

2. Drain the fresh mozzarella balls if necessary.

3. Take a skewer or toothpick and skewer one cherry tomato, followed by a fresh mozzarella ball, and then a fresh basil leaf.

4. Repeat the process until you have assembled the desired number of caprese salad skewers.

5. Arrange the skewers on a serving platter.

6. Drizzle balsamic glaze over the caprese salad skewers just before serving.

7. Enjoy these bite-sized appetizers that showcase the classic flavors of tomatoes, mozzarella, and basil.

Prep time: Approximately 15 minutes

Ingredients:

- 4 chicken breasts

- Juice of 2 lemons

- Zest of 1 lemon

- 3 cloves garlic, minced

- 2 tablespoons fresh herbs (such as rosemary, thyme, or parsley), chopped

- 2 tablespoons olive oil

- Salt and pepper to taste

Preparation:

1. In a bowl, whisk together the lemon juice, lemon zest, minced garlic, chopped fresh herbs, olive oil, salt, and pepper.

2. Place the chicken breasts in a shallow dish or a resealable plastic bag.

3. Pour the marinade over the chicken, making sure it is evenly coated.

4. Cover the dish or seal the bag and marinate the chicken in the refrigerator for at least 30 minutes, or up to overnight for more flavor.

5. Preheat the grill to medium-high heat.

6. Remove the chicken from the marinade and discard the excess marinade.

7. Grill the chicken breasts for about 6-8 minutes per side, or until they reach an internal temperature of 165°F (74°C) and are cooked through.

8. Let the grilled chicken rest for a few minutes before serving.

9. Serve the lemon and herb grilled chicken with your choice of sides, such as roasted vegetables or a salad.

Prep time: Approximately 40 minutes (including marinating time)

Ingredients:

- 1 cup cooked quinoa

- 1 cup mixed vegetables (such as bell peppers, cucumbers, cherry tomatoes, and carrots), chopped

- 1/2 cup chickpeas, rinsed and drained

- 2 tablespoons fresh parsley, chopped

- 2 tablespoons tahini

- Juice of 1 lemon

- 1 tablespoon olive oil

- 1 clove garlic, minced

- Salt and pepper to taste

Preparation:

1. In a bowl, combine the cooked quinoa, mixed vegetables, chickpeas, and fresh parsley.

2. In a separate small bowl, whisk together the tahini, lemon juice, olive oil, minced garlic, salt, and pepper until well combined.

3. Pour the lemon tahini dressing over the quinoa and vegetable mixture.

4. Toss the ingredients together until everything is coated in the dressing.

41

5. Taste and adjust the seasoning if needed.

6. Serve the veggie quinoa bowl as a healthy and satisfying lunch or dinner option.

Prep time: Approximately 15 minutes

Ingredients:

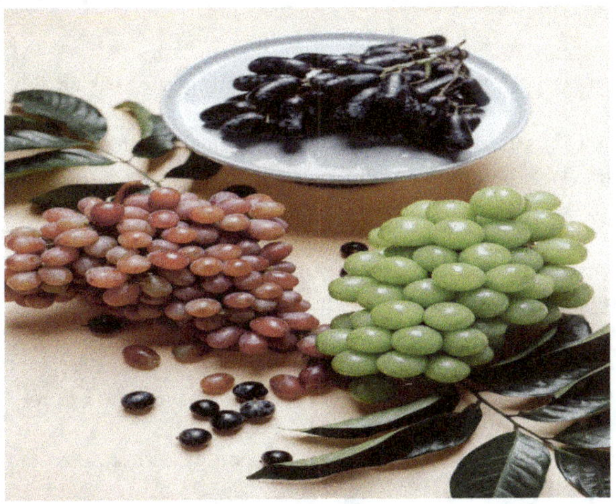

- 2 large sweet potatoes, peeled and cubed

- 1 can black beans, rinsed and drained

- 1 red bell pepper, diced

- 1 small onion, diced

- 2 cloves garlic, minced

- 1 teaspoon ground cumin

- 1 teaspoon chili powder

- Salt and pepper to taste

- 8 small flour tortillas

- 1 cup enchilada sauce

- 1 cup shredded cheddar cheese

- Fresh cilantro for garnish (optional)

Preparation:

1. Preheat the oven to 375°F (190°C) and lightly grease a baking dish.

2. Place the cubed sweet potatoes in a pot of boiling water and cook until tender, about 10 minutes. Drain and set aside.

3. In a large skillet, heat some oil over medium heat. Add the diced red bell pepper, diced onion, minced garlic, ground cumin, chili powder, salt, and pepper. Sauté until the vegetables are softened, about 5 minutes.

4. Add the cooked sweet potatoes and black beans to the skillet. Mash the mixture slightly with a fork or potato masher, leaving some texture.

5. Warm the flour tortillas in the microwave or on a stovetop to make them pliable.

6. Spoon the sweet potato and black bean mixture onto each tortilla, roll them tightly, and place them seam-side down in the greased baking dish.

7. Pour the enchilada sauce over the rolled tortillas, covering them evenly.

8. Sprinkle the shredded cheddar cheese on top.

9. Bake in the preheated oven for about 20-25 minutes, or until the cheese is melted and bubbly.

10. Remove from the oven and let the enchiladas cool slightly.

11. Garnish with fresh cilantro, if desired, and serve the sweet potato and black bean enchiladas as a flavorful and satisfying Mexican-inspired dish.

Prep time: Approximately 1 hour

Ingredients:

- 2 tablespoons olive oil

- 1 onion, chopped

- 3 cloves garlic, minced

- 4 cups diced tomatoes (fresh or canned)

- 1 cup vegetable broth

- 1/2 cup fresh basil leaves, chopped

- Salt and pepper to taste

- Optional toppings: grated Parmesan cheese, croutons, or a drizzle of olive oil

Preparation:

1. Heat the olive oil in a large pot over medium heat.

2. Add the chopped onion and minced garlic to the pot and sauté until the onion is translucent and fragrant.

3. Add the diced tomatoes and vegetable broth to the pot. Bring the mixture to a boil, then reduce the heat and simmer for about 15-20 minutes.

4. Stir in the chopped basil leaves and season with salt and pepper.

5. Use an immersion blender or a regular blender to puree the soup until smooth. Be careful when blending hot liquids.

6. Taste and adjust the seasoning if needed.

7. Ladle the tomato and basil soup into bowls and garnish with your choice of toppings, such as grated Parmesan cheese, croutons, or a drizzle of olive oil.

8. Serve the soup hot and enjoy its comforting flavors.

Prep time: Approximately 30 minutes

Ingredients:

- 1 cup cooked quinoa

- 1 cup cherry tomatoes, halved

- 1 cucumber, diced

- 1/2 red onion, thinly sliced

- 1/2 cup Kalamata olives, pitted and halved

- 1/2 cup crumbled feta cheese

- 1/4 cup fresh parsley, chopped

- Juice of 1 lemon

- 2 tablespoons extra-virgin olive oil

- Salt and pepper to taste

Preparation:

1. In a large bowl, combine the cooked quinoa, cherry tomatoes, diced cucumber, sliced red onion, Kalamata olives, crumbled feta cheese, and chopped parsley.

2. In a small bowl, whisk together the lemon juice, extra-virgin olive oil, salt, and pepper to make the dressing.

3. Pour the dressing over the quinoa salad and toss to coat all the ingredients.

4. Taste and adjust the seasoning if needed.

5. Let the Mediterranean quinoa salad sit for a few minutes to allow the flavors to meld together.

6. Serve the salad as a refreshing and nutritious side dish or light meal.

Prep time: Approximately 20 minutes

Almond Butter and Dark Chocolate Energy Balls:

Ingredients:

- 1 cup rolled oats

- 1/2 cup almond butter

- 1/4 cup honey or maple syrup

- 1/4 cup dark chocolate chips

- 1/4 cup chopped almonds

- 1/4 cup shredded coconut (optional)

- 1 teaspoon vanilla extract

- Pinch of salt

Preparation:

1. In a mixing bowl, combine the rolled oats, almond butter, honey or maple syrup, dark chocolate chips, chopped almonds, shredded coconut (if using), vanilla extract, and a pinch of salt.

2. Stir the ingredients together until well combined.

3. Place the mixture in the refrigerator for about 30 minutes to allow it to firm up slightly.

4. Once chilled, remove the mixture from the refrigerator and roll it into small bite-sized balls using your hands.

5. Repeat the process until all the mixture is used.

6. Store the almond butter and dark chocolate energy balls in an airtight container in the refrigerator for up to one week.

7. Enjoy these energy balls as a healthy and delicious snack whenever you need a quick boost of energy.

Prep time: Approximately 10 minutes

Ingredients:

- 4 salmon fillets

- Juice of 1 lemon

- Juice of 1 orange

- Zest of 1 lemon

- Zest of 1 orange

- 2 cloves garlic, minced

- 2 tablespoons fresh herbs (such as dill, parsley, or thyme), chopped

- 2 tablespoons olive oil

- Salt and pepper to taste

Preparation:

1. Preheat the oven to 375°F (190°C) and line a baking sheet with parchment paper.

2. Place the salmon fillets on the prepared baking sheet.

3. In a bowl, whisk together the lemon juice, orange juice, lemon zest, orange zest, minced garlic, chopped fresh herbs, olive oil, salt, and pepper.

4. Pour the citrus herb marinade over the salmon fillets, making sure they are evenly coated.

5. Let the salmon marinate for about 15-20 minutes to allow the flavors to infuse.

6. Place the baking sheet with the salmon in the preheated oven and bake for approximately 12-15 minutes, or until the salmon is cooked through and flakes easilywith a fork.

7. Remove the salmon from the oven and let it rest for a few minutes before serving.

8. Serve the citrus herb baked salmon as a flavorful and nutritious main dish, accompanied by your choice of sides like roasted vegetables or a fresh salad.

Prep time: Approximately 30 minutes (including marinating time)

Ingredients:

- 2 tablespoons olive oil

- 1 onion, chopped

- 3 cloves garlic, minced

- 4 cups vegetable broth

- 2 cups chopped kale leaves

- 1 can white beans, drained and rinsed

- 1 can diced tomatoes

- 1 teaspoon dried thyme

- 1 teaspoon dried oregano

- Salt and pepper to taste

- Grated Parmesan cheese (optional)

Preparation:

1. Heat the olive oil in a large pot over medium heat.

2. Add the chopped onion and minced garlic to the pot and sauté until the onion is translucent and fragrant.

3. Add the vegetable broth, chopped kale leaves, white beans, diced tomatoes (with their juices), dried thyme, dried oregano, salt, and pepper to the pot.

4. Bring the soup to a boil, then reduce the heat and simmer for about 15-20 minutes, or until the kale is tender.

5. Taste and adjust the seasoning if needed.

6. Ladle the kale and white bean soup into bowls and sprinkle with grated Parmesan cheese, if desired.

7. Serve the soup hot and enjoy its comforting and nourishing qualities.

Prep time: Approximately 30 minutes

Ingredients:

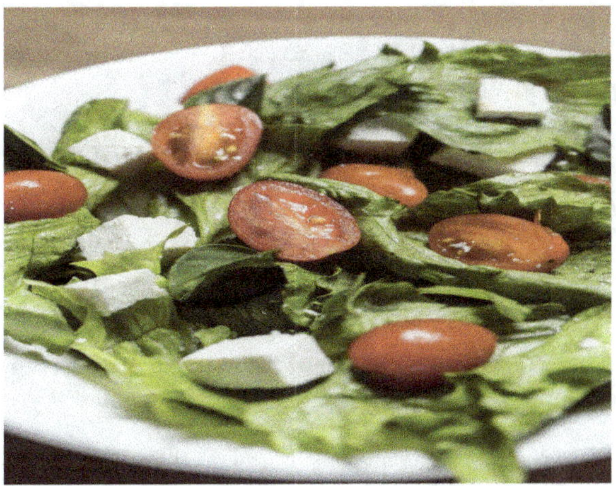

- 1 cup orzo pasta

- 1 cup cherry tomatoes, halved

- 1 cucumber, diced

- 1/2 red onion, thinly sliced

- 1/2 cup Kalamata olives, pitted and halved

- 1/2 cup crumbled feta cheese

- 1/4 cup fresh parsley, chopped

- Juice of 1 lemon

- 2 tablespoons extra-virgin olive oil

- Salt and pepper to taste

Preparation:

1. Cook the orzo pasta according to the package instructions. Drain and let it cool.

2. In a large bowl, combine the cooked orzo pasta, cherry tomatoes, diced cucumber, sliced red onion, Kalamata olives, crumbled feta cheese, and chopped parsley.

3. In a small bowl, whisk together the lemon juice, extra-virgin olive oil, salt, and pepper to make the dressing.

4. Pour the dressing over the orzo salad and toss to coat all the ingredients.

5. Taste and adjust the seasoning if needed.

6. Let the Greek orzo salad sit for a few minutes to allow the flavors to meld together.

7. Serve the salad as a refreshing and flavorful side dish or light meal.

Prep time: Approximately 20 minutes

Garlic Herb Roasted Vegetables:

Ingredients:

- Assorted vegetables of your choice (e.g., carrots, bell peppers, zucchini, broccoli, cauliflower, etc.), cut into bite-sized pieces

- 3 tablespoons olive oil

- 3 cloves garlic, minced

- 1 teaspoon dried thyme

- 1 teaspoon dried rosemary

- Salt and pepper to taste

Preparation:

1. Preheat the oven to 425°F (220°C) and line a baking sheet with parchment paper.

2. In a large bowl, combine the assorted vegetables, olive oil, minced garlic, dried thyme, dried rosemary, salt, and pepper. Toss until the vegetables are evenly coated with the seasonings.

3. Spread the vegetables in a single layer on the prepared baking sheet.

4. Roast the vegetables in the preheated oven for about 20-25 minutes, or until they are tender and slightly caramelized, stirring once or twice during cooking.

5. Remove the roasted vegetables from the oven and let them cool slightly before serving.

6. Serve the garlic herb roasted vegetables as a delicious and healthy side dish to complement any meal.

Prep time: Approximately 30 minutes

Ingredients:

- 2 boneless, skinless chicken breasts, cut into thin strips

- 2 tablespoons coconut oil

- 1 onion, sliced

- 2 cloves garlic, minced

- 1 red bell pepper, sliced

- 1 yellow bell pepper, sliced

- 1 cup broccoli florets

- 1 cup snap peas

- 1 can coconut milk

- 2 tablespoons red curry paste

- 1 tablespoon soy sauce

- 1 tablespoon fish sauce (optional)

- Juice of 1 lime

- Fresh cilantro for garnish (optional)

- Cooked rice or noodles for serving

Preparation:

1. Heat the coconut oil in a large skillet or wok over medium-high heat.

2. Add the chicken strips to the skillet and cook until they are browned and cooked through. Remove the cooked chicken from the skillet and set it aside.

3. In the same skillet, add the sliced onion and minced garlic. Sauté for a few minutes until the onion becomes translucent and fragrant.

4. Add the sliced bell peppers, broccoli florets, and snap peas to the skillet. Stir-fry for about 5 minutes, or until the vegetables are crisp-tender.

5. In a bowl, whisk together the coconut milk, red curry paste, soy sauce, fish sauce (if using), and lime juice.

6. Pour the coconut curry sauce into the skillet with the vegetables. Stir well to combine.

7. Return the cooked chicken to the skillet and toss it with the vegetables and sauce until everything is coated evenly.

8. Cook for another 2-3 minutes, or until the chicken is heated through and the flavors have melded together.

9. Remove the skillet from the heat and garnish the coconut curry chicken stir-fry with fresh cilantro, if desired.

10. Serve the stir-fry over cooked rice or noodles for a satisfying and flavorful meal.

Prep time: Approximately 30 minutes

Ingredients:

- 1 cup frozen mixed berries (such as strawberries, blueberries, and raspberries)

- 1 ripe banana

- 1 cup fresh spinach leaves

- 1/2 cup almond milk or any other milk of your choice

- 1 tablespoon honey or maple syrup (optional)

- Toppings: sliced fresh berries, granola, sliced almonds, chia seeds,shredded coconut, etc.

Preparation:

1. In a blender, combine the frozen mixed berries, ripe banana, fresh spinach leaves, almond milk, and honey or maple syrup (if using).

2. Blend the ingredients until smooth and creamy. If the mixture is too thick, you can add a little more almond milk to thin it out.

3. Pour the smoothie into a bowl.

4. Top the smoothie bowl with your desired toppings, such as sliced fresh berries, granola, sliced almonds, chia seeds, shredded coconut, or any other toppings you prefer.

5. Enjoy the berry spinach smoothie bowl immediately with a spoon for a nutritious and refreshing breakfast or snack.

Prep time: Approximately 5 minutes

Ingredients:

- 2 cans chickpeas, drained and rinsed

- 1/4 cup fresh lemon juice

- 1/4 cup tahini

- 3 cloves garlic, roasted

- 2 tablespoons extra-virgin olive oil

- 1 teaspoon ground cumin

- 1/2 teaspoon salt

- 2-4 tablespoons water (as needed)

- Optional toppings: extra olive oil, paprika, chopped fresh parsley

Preparation:

1. Preheat the oven to 400°F (200°C).

2. Slice off the top portion of the garlic bulb to expose the cloves. Drizzle with a little olive oil, wrap it in foil, and roast it in the preheated oven for about 30 minutes, or until the garlic becomes soft and golden.

3. In a food processor, combine the drained and rinsed chickpeas, fresh lemon juice, tahini, roasted garlic cloves, extra-virgin olive oil, ground cumin, and salt.

4. Process the mixture until smooth and creamy. If the hummus seems too thick, you can add water, one tablespoon at a time, until you reach your desired consistency.

5. Taste the hummus and adjust the seasoning if needed, adding more salt or lemon juice according to your preference.

6. Transfer the roasted garlic hummus to a serving bowl.

7. Optional: Drizzle some extra olive oil over the hummus and sprinkle with paprika and chopped fresh parsley for added flavor and presentation.

8. Serve the roasted garlic hummus with pita bread, vegetable sticks, or as a spread for sandwiches and wraps.

Prep time: Approximately 40 minutes (including roasting garlic)

Ingredients:

For the falafel:

- 2 cans chickpeas, drained and rinsed

- 1/2 cup fresh parsley, chopped

- 1/2 cup fresh cilantro, chopped

- 1 small onion, chopped

- 3 cloves garlic, minced

- 2 tablespoons olive oil

- 2 tablespoons all-purpose flour

- 2 teaspoons ground cumin

- 1 teaspoon ground coriander

- 1/2 teaspoon baking soda

- Salt and pepper to taste

For the tzatziki sauce:

- 1 cup Greek yogurt

- 1/2 cucumber, finely diced

- 1 clove garlic, minced

- 1 tablespoon fresh dill, chopped

- 1 tablespoon fresh lemon juice

- Salt and pepper to taste

Preparation:

1. Preheat the oven to 375°F (190°C) and line a baking sheet with parchment paper.

2. In a food processor, combine the drained and rinsed chickpeas, fresh parsley, fresh cilantro, chopped onion, minced garlic, olive oil, all-purpose flour, ground cumin, ground coriander, baking soda, salt, and pepper.

3. Pulse the ingredients until a coarse mixture forms. Be careful not to over-process; you want the mixture to have some texture.

4. Shape the falafel mixture into small patties or balls and place them on the prepared baking sheet.

5. Bake the falafel in the preheated oven for about 20-25 minutes, or until they are golden brown and crispy on the outside.

6. While the falafel is baking, prepare the tzatziki sauce. In a bowl, combine the Greek yogurt, finely diced cucumber, minced garlic, fresh dill, fresh lemon juice, salt, and pepper. Mix well to combine.

7. Once the falafel is cooked, remove them from the oven and let them cool slightly.

8. Serve the baked falafel with the tzatziki sauce as a delicious vegetarian main course or as a filling for pita bread or wraps.

Prep time: Approximately 45 minutes

Quinoa Stuffed Portobello Mushrooms:

Ingredients:

- 4 large Portobello mushrooms

- 1 cup cooked quinoa

- 1/2 cup diced bell peppers (any color)

- 1/2 cup diced zucchini

- 1/2 cup diced onion

- 2 cloves garlic, minced

- 1 tablespoon olive oil

- 1/2 teaspoon dried thyme

- 1/2 teaspoon dried oregano

- Salt and pepper to taste

- Grated Parmesan cheese (optional, for topping)

Preparation:

1. Preheat the oven to 375°F (190°C) and lightly grease a baking dish.

2. Remove the stems from the Portobello mushrooms and gently scrape out the gills using a spoon.

3. In a skillet, heat the olive oil over medium heat. Add the diced bell peppers, diced zucchini, diced onion, and minced garlic. Sauté for a few minutes until the vegetables are tender.

4. Stir in the cooked quinoa, dried thyme, dried oregano, salt, and pepper. Cook for an additional 2-3 minutes, allowing the flavors to blend.

5. Spoon the quinoa mixture into the hollowed-out Portobello mushrooms, pressing it down gently.

6. Place the stuffed mushrooms in the greased baking dish and sprinkle grated Parmesan cheese on top, if desired.

7. Bake the stuffed mushrooms in the preheated oven for about 20-25 minutes, or until the mushrooms are tender and the cheese is melted and golden.

8. Remove the stuffed mushrooms from the oven and let them cool for a few minutes before serving.

9. Serve the quinoa stuffed Portobello mushrooms as a flavorful and satisfying vegetarian main course or as a hearty side dish.

Prep time: Approximately 30 minutes

Lemon Poppy Seed Pancakes:

Ingredients:

- 1 cup all-purpose flour

- 2 tablespoons granulated sugar

- 1 tablespoon poppy seeds

- 1 teaspoon baking powder

- 1/2 teaspoon baking soda

- 1/4 teaspoon salt

- 1 cup buttermilk

- 1 large egg

- 2 tablespoons unsalted butter, melted

- Zest of 1 lemon

- Juice of 1/2 lemon

- Cooking spray or additional butter for greasing the pan

Preparation:

1. In a large bowl, whisk together the all-purpose flour, granulated sugar, poppy seeds, baking powder, baking soda, and salt.

2. In a separate bowl, whisk together the buttermilk, egg, melted butter, lemon zest, and lemon juice.

3. Pour the wet ingredients into the dry ingredients and stir until just combined.4. Let the pancake batter rest for about 5-10 minutes.

5. Preheat a non-stick skillet or griddle over medium heat and lightly grease it with cooking spray or butter.

6. Pour 1/4 cup of the pancake batter onto the preheated skillet for each pancake. Cook until bubbles form on the surface, then flip and cook for an additional 1-2 minutes, or until golden brown.

7. Repeat with the remaining batter, adding more cooking spray or butter as needed.

8. Serve the lemon poppy seed pancakes warm with your favorite toppings, such as maple syrup, fresh berries, or a dusting of powdered sugar.

Prep time: Approximately 20 minutes

Ingredients:

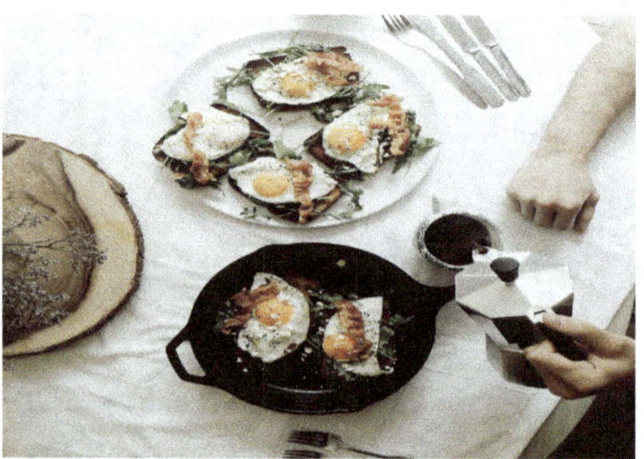

- 1 bunch asparagus, woody ends trimmed

- 2 tablespoons olive oil

- Salt and pepper to taste

- 1/4 cup grated Parmesan cheese

Preparation:

1. Preheat the oven to 425°F (220°C) and line a baking sheet with parchment paper.

2. Place the trimmed asparagus on the prepared baking sheet and drizzle with olive oil. Toss the asparagus to coat evenly with the oil.

3. Season the asparagus with salt and pepper to taste, then sprinkle the grated Parmesan cheese over the top.

4. Roast the asparagus in the preheated oven for about 10-12 minutes, or until the asparagus is tender and the cheese is melted and lightly browned.

5. Remove the roasted asparagus from the oven and serve it as a delicious and healthy side dish.

Prep time: Approximately 15 minutes

Ingredients:

- 4 large flour tortillas

- 1 ripe avocado, sliced

- 1 cup canned black beans, rinsed and drained

- 1 cup shredded cheese (such as cheddar, Monterey Jack, or Mexican blend)

- 1/4 cup chopped fresh cilantro

- 1/4 cup diced red onion

- 1/4 cup diced tomatoes

- Salt and pepper to taste

- Cooking spray or oil for cooking

Preparation:

1. Lay out two of the flour tortillas on a clean surface.

2. Divide the sliced avocado, black beans, shredded cheese, chopped cilantro, diced red onion, and diced tomatoes evenly between the two tortillas.

3. Season with salt and pepper to taste.

4. Place the remaining two tortillas on top of the filling to create quesadillas.

5. Preheat a large skillet or griddle over medium heat and lightly grease it with cooking spray or oil.

6. Carefully transfer one quesadilla to the preheated skillet and cook for about 2-3 minutes on each side, or until the tortilla is golden brown and the cheese is melted.

7. Repeat with the second quesadilla.

8. Remove the quesadillas from the skillet and let them cool for a minute before slicing into wedges.

9. Serve the avocado and black bean quesadillas as a tasty and satisfying vegetarian meal. They can be enjoyed on their own or served with salsa, guacamole, or sour cream.

Prep time: Approximately 15 minutes

Chapter 4:

SHARPENING FOCUS AND CONCENTRATION

Green Tea and Matcha Smoothie:

Ingredients:

- 1 cup brewed green tea, chilled

- 1 ripe banana

- 1 cup spinach

- 1 tablespoon matcha powder

- 1/2 cup Greek yogurt

- 1 tablespoon honey or maple syrup (optional, for sweetness)

- Ice cubes (optional)

Preparation:

1. In a blender, combine the brewed green tea, ripe banana, spinach, matcha powder, Greek yogurt, and honey or maple syrup (if desired).

2. Blend on high speed until the ingredients are well combined and the smoothie is creamy.

3. If desired, add a few ice cubes and blend again until the smoothie is chilled.

4. Pour the green tea and matcha smoothie into glasses and serve immediately as a refreshing and nutritious beverage.

Prep time: Approximately 5 minutes

Ingredients:

For the salad:

- 1 cup cooked quinoa

- 2 cups chopped kale leaves

- 1 cup cherry tomatoes, halved

- 1/2 cup diced cucumber

- 1/4 cup diced red onion

- 1/4 cup crumbled feta cheese (optional)

- 1/4 cup chopped fresh parsley

- Salt and pepper to taste

For the lemon vinaigrette:

- 3 tablespoons fresh lemon juice

- 1/4 cup extra virgin olive oil

- 1 clove garlic, minced

- 1 teaspoon Dijon mustard

- Salt and pepper to taste

Preparation:

1. In a large bowl, combine the cooked quinoa, chopped kale leaves, cherry tomatoes, diced cucumber, diced red onion, crumbled feta cheese (if using), and chopped fresh parsley.

2. Season the salad with salt and pepper to taste.

3. In a separate small bowl, whisk together the fresh lemon juice, extra virgin olive oil, minced garlic, Dijon mustard, salt, and pepper to make the lemon vinaigrette.

4. Drizzle the lemon vinaigrette over the quinoa and kale salad and toss gently to coat the ingredients evenly.

5. Let the salad sit for a few minutes to allow the flavors to meld together.

6. Serve the quinoa and kale salad as a nutritious and flavorful side dish or as a light and satisfying main course.

Prep time: Approximately 15 minutes

Ingredients:

- 4 salmon fillets

- 2 tablespoons olive oil

- 2 tablespoons fresh lemon juice

- Zest of 1 lemon

- 2 cloves garlic, minced

- 1 tablespoon chopped fresh dill

- 1 tablespoon chopped fresh parsley

- Salt and pepper to taste

Preparation:

1. Preheat the oven to 375°F (190°C) and line a baking sheet with parchment paper.

2. Place the salmon fillets on the prepared baking sheet.

3. In a small bowl, whisk together the olive oil, fresh lemon juice, lemon zest, minced garlic, chopped fresh dill, chopped fresh parsley, salt, and pepper.

4. Drizzle the lemon herb mixture over the salmon fillets, making sure to coat them evenly.

5. Bake the salmon in the preheated oven for about 10-12 minutes, or until the fish is cooked through and flakes easily with a fork.

6. Remove the baked salmon from the oven and let it rest for a few minutes before serving.

7. Serve the lemon herb baked salmon as a delicious and healthy main course, accompanied by steamed vegetables or a side salad.

Prep time: Approximately 20 minutes

Cauliflower Fried Rice:

Ingredients:

- 1 small head cauliflower, riced (using a food processor or grater)

- 2 tablespoons sesame oil

- 1 small onion, diced

- 2 cloves garlic, minced

- 1 cup diced carrots

- 1 cup frozen peas

- 2 eggs, lightly beaten

- 3 tablespoons soy sauce (or tamari for a gluten-free option)

- 1 tablespoon oyster sauce (optional)

- Salt and pepper to taste

- Sliced green onions and sesame seeds for garnish

Preparation:

1. Heat the sesame oil in a large skillet or wok over medium heat.

2. Add the diced onion and minced garlic to the skillet and sauté until fragrant and translucent.

3. Add the diced carrots and frozen peas to the skillet and cook for a few minutes until the vegetables are tender.

4. Push the vegetables to one side of the skillet and pour the beaten eggs into the cleared space. Scramble the eggs until cooked through.

5. Add the riced cauliflower to the skillet and stir to combine with the cooked vegetables and eggs.

6. Stir in the soy sauce and oyster sauce (if using), and season with salt and pepper to taste.

7. Cook the cauliflower fried rice foran additional 5-7 minutes, stirring occasionally, until the cauliflower is tender but still slightly crisp.

8. Remove the skillet from heat and garnish the cauliflower fried rice with sliced green onions and sesame seeds.

9. Serve the cauliflower fried rice as a healthier alternative to traditional fried rice, packed with vegetables and delicious flavors.

Prep time: Approximately 20 minutes

Ingredients:

- 1 cup dried lentils (green or brown), rinsed and drained

- 1 tablespoon olive oil

- 1 onion, diced

- 2 carrots, diced

- 2 celery stalks, diced

- 2 cloves garlic, minced

- 1 can (14 oz) diced tomatoes

- 4 cups vegetable broth

- 2 cups water

- 1 teaspoon dried thyme

- 1 teaspoon dried oregano

- Salt and pepper to taste

- Fresh parsley for garnish (optional)

Preparation:

1. In a large pot, heat the olive oil over medium heat.

2. Add the diced onion, carrots, celery, and minced garlic to the pot. Sauté until the vegetables are tender.

3. Add the rinsed lentils, diced tomatoes (with their juice), vegetable broth, water, dried thyme, and dried oregano to the pot. Stir to combine.

4. Bring the soup to a boil, then reduce the heat to low and let it simmer for about 30-40 minutes, or until the lentils are cooked and tender.

5. Season the lentil and vegetable soup with salt and pepper to taste.

6. Ladle the soup into bowls and garnish with fresh parsley, if desired.

7. Serve the lentil and vegetable soup as a hearty and nutritious meal, accompanied by crusty bread or a side salad.

Prep time: Approximately 45 minutes

Greek Yogurt and Berry Parfait:

Ingredients:

- 1 cup Greek yogurt

- 1 cup mixed berries (such as strawberries, blueberries, raspberries)

- 1/4 cup granola

- 1 tablespoon honey or maple syrup (optional, for sweetness)

- Fresh mint leaves for garnish (optional)

Preparation:

1. In a glass or serving dish, layer half of the Greek yogurt.

2. Add a layer of mixed berries on top of the yogurt.

3. Sprinkle a layer of granola over the berries.

4. Repeat the layers with the remaining Greek yogurt, mixed berries, and granola.

5. Drizzle honey or maple syrup over the top, if desired, for added sweetness.

6. Garnish with fresh mint leaves, if desired, for a pop of freshness.

7. Serve the Greek yogurt and berry parfait as a delicious and nutritious breakfast or dessert option.

Prep time: Approximately 5 minutes

Garlic Herb Roasted Chicken:

Ingredients:

- 4 bone-in, skin-on chicken thighs

- 2 tablespoons olive oil

- 4 cloves garlic, minced

- 1 teaspoon dried rosemary

- 1 teaspoon dried thyme

- 1 teaspoon dried oregano

- Salt and pepper to taste

- Lemon wedges for serving (optional)

Preparation:

1. Preheat the oven to 400°F (200°C) and line a baking sheet with parchment paper.

2. In a small bowl, combine the olive oil, minced garlic, dried rosemary, dried thyme, dried oregano, salt, and pepper.

3. Place the chicken thighs on the prepared baking sheet and rub them with the garlic herb mixture, making sure to coat them evenly.

4. Roast the chicken in the preheated oven for about 35-40 minutes, or until the chicken is golden brown and cooked through.

5. Remove the roasted chicken from the oven and let it rest for a few minutes before serving.

6. Serve the garlic herb roasted chicken with lemon wedges on the side, if desired, for a burst of citrus flavor.

Prep time: Approximately 10 minutes | Cook time: Approximately 35-40 minutes

Ingredients:

- 12 large button mushrooms, stems removed

- 1 tablespoon olive oil

- 2 cups fresh spinach, chopped

- 1/2 cup crumbled feta cheese

- 2 cloves garlic, minced

- Salt and pepper to taste

Preparation:

1. Preheat the oven to 375°F (190°C) and line a baking sheet with parchment paper.

2. Place the mushroom caps on the prepared baking sheet, rounded side down.

3. Heat the olive oil in a skillet over medium heat. Add the chopped spinach and minced garlic, and sauté until the spinach is wilted.

4. Remove the skillet from heat and let the spinach mixture cool slightly.

5. In a bowl, combine the sautéed spinach, crumbled feta cheese, salt, and pepper.

6. Spoon the spinach and feta mixture into the mushroom caps, filling them generously.

7. Bake the stuffed mushrooms in the preheated oven for about 15-20 minutes, or until the mushrooms are tender and the filling is golden brown.

8. Remove the stuffed mushrooms from the oven and let them cool for a few minutes before serving.

9. Serve the spinach and feta stuffed mushrooms as a flavorful and satisfying appetizer or side dish.

Prep time: Approximately 15 minutes | Cook time: Approximately 15-20 minutes

Chia Seed Energy Bars:

Ingredients:

- 1 cup pitted dates

- 1 cup nuts of your choice (e.g., almonds, cashews, walnuts)

- 1/4 cup chia seeds

- 1/4 cup unsweetened shredded coconut

- 2 tablespoons honey or maple syrup

- 1 teaspoon vanilla extract

Preparation:

1. Place the pitted dates in a food processor and process until they form a sticky paste.

2. Add the nuts to the processor and pulse until they are finely chopped and combined with the dates.

3. Transfer the date and nut mixture to a bowl and stir in the chia seeds, shredded coconut, honey or maple syrup, and vanilla extract. Mix well until all the ingredients are evenly combined.

4. Line a baking dish or pan with parchment paper.

5. Press the mixture firmly into the prepared baking dish, using the back of a spoon or your hands to flatten it evenly.

6. Refrigerate the mixture for at least 1-2 hours, or until it becomes firm.

7. Remove the chilled mixture from the refrigerator and cut it into bars or squares of your desired size.

8. Store the chia seed energy bars in an airtight container in the refrigerator for up to 1 week.

9. Enjoy the chia seed energy barsas a healthy and convenient snack option on the go.

Prep time: Approximately 15 minutes | Chill time: Approximately 1-2 hours

Ingredients:

- 2 cups cooked chickpeas (or 1 can, drained and rinsed)

- 2 tablespoons olive oil

- 1 teaspoon ground turmeric

- 1/2 teaspoon ground cumin

- 1/2 teaspoon paprika

- 1/2 teaspoon salt (adjust to taste)

- Fresh cilantro or parsley for garnish (optional)

Preparation:

1. Preheat the oven to 400°F (200°C) and line a baking sheet with parchment paper.

2. In a bowl, combine the cooked chickpeas, olive oil, ground turmeric, ground cumin, paprika, and salt. Toss well to coat the chickpeas evenly with the spices.

3. Spread the seasoned chickpeas in a single layer on the prepared baking sheet.

4. Roast the chickpeas in the preheated oven for about 25-30 minutes, or until they are golden brown and crispy, stirring once or twice during cooking.

5. Remove the roasted chickpeas from the oven and let them cool slightly.

6. Garnish with fresh cilantro or parsley, if desired, for added freshness and flavor.

7. Serve the turmeric roasted chickpeas as a crunchy and flavorful snack or use them as a topping for salads or bowls.

Prep time: Approximately 5 minutes | Cook time: Approximately 25-30 minutes

Ingredients:

- 2 boneless, skinless chicken breasts

- 1 tablespoon olive oil

- 1 teaspoon dried oregano

- Salt and pepper to taste

- 4 cups mixed salad greens

- 1 cup cherry tomatoes, halved

- 1 cucumber, sliced

- 1/2 red onion, thinly sliced

- 1/2 cup Kalamata olives

- 1/2 cup crumbled feta cheese

- 2 tablespoons lemon juice

- 2 tablespoons extra virgin olive oil

- 1 teaspoon dried oregano

Preparation:

1. Preheat the grill or grill pan over medium-high heat.

2. Drizzle the chicken breasts with olive oil and season them with dried oregano, salt, and pepper.

3. Grill the chicken for about 6-7 minutes per side, or until cooked through. Let it rest for a few minutes, then slice it into strips.

4. In a large salad bowl, combine the mixed salad greens, cherry tomatoes, cucumber slices, red onion, Kalamata olives, and crumbled feta cheese.

5. In a small bowl, whisk together the lemon juice, extra virgin olive oil, dried oregano, salt, and pepper to make the dressing.

6. Pour the dressing over the salad ingredients and toss gently to combine.

7. Divide the salad onto plates and top each serving with grilled chicken slices.

8. Serve the Greek salad with grilled chicken as a light and refreshing main course.

Prep time: Approximately 15 minutes | Cook time: Approximately 15 minutes

Baked Cod with Tomato and Basil:

Ingredients:

- 4 cod fillets

- 2 tablespoons olive oil

- 2 cloves garlic, minced

- 1 cup cherry tomatoes, halved

- 1/4 cup chopped fresh basil

- Salt and pepper to taste

- Lemon wedges for serving (optional)

Preparation:

1. Preheat the oven to 400°F (200°C) and line a baking dish with parchment paper.

2. Place the cod fillets in the prepared baking dish.

3. In a small bowl, mix together the olive oil, minced garlic, cherry tomatoes, chopped basil, salt, and pepper.

4. Spoon the tomato and basil mixture over the cod fillets, covering them evenly.

5. Bake the cod in the preheated oven for about 15-20 minutes, or until the fish is opaque and flakes easily with a fork.

6. Remove the baked cod from the oven and let it rest for a few minutes before serving.

7. Serve the baked cod with tomato and basil, accompanied by lemon wedges if desired, for a burst of citrus flavor.

Prep time: Approximately 10 minutes | Cook time: Approximately 15-20 minutes

Berry Chia Seed Pudding:

Ingredients:

- 1/4 cup chia seeds

- 1 cup almond milk (or any milk of your choice)

- 1 tablespoon honey or maple syrup

- 1/2 teaspoon vanilla extract

- 1/2 cup mixed berries (such as strawberries, blueberries, raspberries)

- Fresh mint leaves for garnish (optional)

Preparation:

1. In a bowl, combine the chia seeds, almond milk, honey or maple syrup, and vanilla extract. Stir well to combine.

2. Let the mixture sit for about 5 minutes, then stir again to prevent clumping.

3. Cover the bowl and refrigerate the chia seed mixture for at least 2 hours or overnight, allowing it to thicken.

4. Once the chia seed pudding has thickened, give it a good stir to break up any clumps.

5. In serving glasses or bowls, layer the chia seed pudding with mixed berries.

6. Garnish with fresh mint leaves, if desired, for added freshness and presentation.

7. Serve the berry chia seed pudding as a healthy and satisfying breakfast or dessert option.

Prep time: Approximately 5 minutes | Chill time: Approximately 2 hours or overnight

Caprese Quinoa Stuffed Peppers:

Ingredients:

- 4 bell peppers (any color)

- 1 cup cooked quinoa

- 1 cup cherry tomatoes, halved

- 1 cup fresh mozzarella balls, halved

- 1/4 cup chopped fresh basil

- 2 tablespoons balsamic glaze

- Salt and pepper to taste

Preparation:

1. Preheat the oven to 375°F (190°C) and line a baking dish with parchment paper.

2. Cut the tops off the bell peppers and remove the seeds and membranes from the inside.

3. In a bowl, combine the cooked quinoa, cherry tomatoes, fresh mozzarella, chopped basil, balsamic glaze, salt, and pepper. Mix well.

4. Spoon the quinoa mixture into the hollowed-out bell peppersfrom step 3.

5. Place the stuffed bell peppers in the prepared baking dish.

6. Bake in the preheated oven for about 25-30 minutes, or until the peppers are tender and the filling is heated through.

7. Remove the stuffed peppers from the oven and let them cool for a few minutes before serving.

8. Serve the caprese quinoa stuffed peppers as a flavorful and nutritious vegetarian main course or side dish.

Prep time: Approximately 20 minutes | Cook time: Approximately 25-30 minutes

Roasted Garlic White Bean Dip:

Ingredients:

- 1 can (15 ounces) white beans (such as cannellini beans), drained and rinsed

- 3 cloves garlic, roasted

- 2 tablespoons lemon juice

- 2 tablespoons extra virgin olive oil

- 1/4 teaspoon cumin

- Salt and pepper to taste

- Fresh parsley or chives for garnish (optional)

- Assorted vegetables, pita chips, or crackers for serving

Preparation:

1. Preheat the oven to 400°F (200°C).

2. Slice off the top of each garlic clove to expose the cloves. Place the cloves on a sheet of aluminum foil, drizzle with olive oil, and wrap tightly. Roast the garlic in the preheated oven for about 20-25 minutes, or until soft and golden.

3. In a food processor or blender, combine the white beans, roasted garlic cloves, lemon juice, olive oil, cumin, salt, and pepper.

4. Process the ingredients until smooth and creamy, scraping down the sides as needed.

5. Taste the dip and adjust the seasoning if desired.

6. Transfer the roasted garlic white bean dip to a serving bowl and garnish with fresh parsley or chives, if desired.

7. Serve the dip with assorted vegetables, pita chips, or crackers for a delicious and healthy appetizer or snack.

Prep time: Approximately 5 minutes | Cook time: Approximately 20-25 minutes for roasting garlic

Quinoa and Black Bean Salad:

Ingredients:

- 1 cup cooked quinoa

- 1 can (15 ounces) black beans, drained and rinsed

- 1 red bell pepper, diced

- 1 cup corn kernels (fresh or frozen)

- 1/4 cup chopped fresh cilantro

- 2 green onions, sliced

- Juice of 1 lime

- 2 tablespoons extra virgin olive oil

- 1 teaspoon ground cumin

- Salt and pepper to taste

- Optional toppings: diced avocado, crumbled feta cheese, chopped tomatoes

Preparation:

1. In a large bowl, combine the cooked quinoa, black beans, diced red bell pepper, corn kernels, chopped cilantro, and sliced green onions.

2. In a small bowl, whisk together the lime juice, olive oil, ground cumin, salt, and pepper to make the dressing.

3. Pour the dressing over the quinoa and black bean mixture, and toss gently to coat all the ingredients.

4. Taste and adjust the seasoning if needed.

5. If desired, add diced avocado, crumbled feta cheese, or chopped tomatoes as additional toppings.

6. Serve the quinoa and black bean salad as a satisfying and protein-rich side dish or light lunch.

Prep time: Approximately 15 minutes | Cook time: Varies depending on quinoa cooking time

Ingredients:

- 2 cups all-purpose flour

- 3/4 cup granulated sugar

- 2 teaspoons baking powder

- 1/2 teaspoon baking soda

- 1/4 teaspoon salt

- Zest of 2 lemons

- 1/4 cup lemon juice

- 1/2 cup unsalted butter, melted

- 2/3 cup milk

- 2 large eggs

- 1 tablespoon poppy seeds

Preparation:

1. Preheat the oven to 375°F (190°C) and line a muffin tin with paper liners.

2. In a large bowl, whisk together the flour, sugar, baking powder, baking soda, salt, and lemon zest.

3. In a separate bowl, mix together the lemon juice, melted butter, milk, and eggs until well combined.

4. Pour the wet ingredients into the dry ingredients and stir until just combined. Do not overmix.

5. Gently fold in the poppy seeds.

6. Divide the batter evenly among the muffin cups, filling each about 2/3 full.

7. Bake in the preheated oven for approximately 18-20 minutes, or until a toothpick inserted into the center of a muffin comes out clean.

8. Remove the muffins from the oven and let them cool in the pan for a few minutes before transferring them to a wire rack to cool completely.

9. Enjoy the lemon poppy seed muffins as a delightful treat for breakfast or snack time.

Prep time: Approximately 15 minutes | Bake time: Approximately 18-20 minutes

Ingredients:

- 2 medium zucchini

- 1/2 cup breadcrumbs

- 1/4 cup grated Parmesan cheese

- 1 teaspoon dried Italian seasoning

- 1/2 teaspoon garlic powder

- Salt and pepper to taste

- 2 large eggs, lightly beaten

- Cooking spray or olive oil for greasing

Preparation:

1. Preheat the oven to 425°F (220°C) and line a baking sheet with parchment paper or lightly grease it with cooking spray or olive oil.

2. Cut the zucchini into long, thin strips resembling fries.

3. In a shallow dish, combine the breadcrumbs, grated Parmesan cheese, dried Italian seasoning, garlic powder, salt, and pepper.

4. Dip each zucchini strip into the beaten eggs, allowing any excess to drip off, then coat it in the breadcrumb mixture, pressing gently to adhere the breadcrumbs.

5. Place the coated zucchini fries on the prepared baking sheet, spacing them apart.

6. Bake in the preheated oven for about 15-20 minutes, or until the zucchini fries are golden and crispy.

7. Remove the baked zucchini fries from the oven and let them cool for a few minutes before serving.

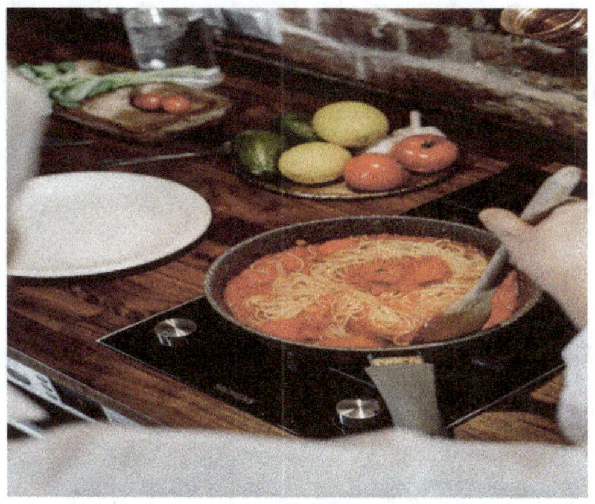

8. Serve the zucchini fries as a healthier alternative to traditional fries, accompanied by a dipping sauce of your choice.

Prep time: Approximately 15 minutes | Bake time: Approximately 15-20 minutes

Spinach and Mushroom Quiche:

Ingredients:

- 1 pre-made pie crust

- 1 tablespoon olive oil

- 1 small onion, finely chopped

- 8 ounces mushrooms, sliced

- 2 cups fresh spinach leaves

- 4 large eggs

- 1 cup milk (whole or reduced fat)

- 1/2 cup shredded cheese (such as cheddar or Swiss)

- Salt and pepper to taste

- Optional: additional herbs orseasonings of your choice (e.g., thyme, garlic powder)

Preparation:

1. Preheat the oven to 375°F (190°C) and place the pre-made pie crust in a pie dish or tart pan. Set aside.

2. In a skillet, heat the olive oil over medium heat. Add the chopped onion and sliced mushrooms, and sauté until the mushrooms are browned and the onions are translucent.

3. Add the fresh spinach leaves to the skillet and cook until wilted. Remove from heat and set aside.

4. In a mixing bowl, whisk together the eggs, milk, shredded cheese, salt, pepper, and any additional herbs or seasonings you prefer.

5. Spread the sautéed mushroom, onion, and spinach mixture evenly over the bottom of the pie crust.

6. Pour the egg mixture over the vegetables, ensuring that it is evenly distributed.

7. Place the quiche in the preheated oven and bake for approximately 30-35 minutes, or until the center is set and the top is golden.

8. Remove the quiche from the oven and let it cool for a few minutes before slicing and serving.

9. Enjoy the spinach and mushroom quiche as a delicious brunch or lunch option.

Prep time: Approximately 20 minutes | Bake time: Approximately 30-35 minutes

Ingredients:

- 4 nori seaweed sheets

- 2 cups sushi rice, cooked and seasoned

- 1 ripe avocado, sliced

- 1/2 cucumber, cut into thin strips

- Soy sauce, for dipping

- Pickled ginger, for serving

- Wasabi, for serving (optional)

Preparation:

1. Lay a bamboo sushi mat on a clean surface and place a nori seaweed sheet on top.

2. Wet your hands with water to prevent the rice from sticking. Take a handful of sushi rice and spread it evenly over the nori sheet, leaving a small border at the top.

3. Place avocado slices and cucumber strips horizontally across the middle of the rice.

4. Using the bamboo mat, roll the sushi tightly from the bottom, applying gentle pressure to shape it.

5. Wet the border of the nori sheet with water to seal the roll.

6. Repeat the process with the remaining nori sheets and ingredients.

7. Using a sharp knife, slice each sushi roll into bite-sized pieces.

8. Serve the avocado and cucumber sushi rolls with soy sauce for dipping, along with pickled ginger and wasabi if desired.

9. Enjoy the homemade sushi rolls as a tasty and refreshing snack or light meal.

Prep time: Approximately 30 minutes (excluding sushi rice cooking time) | Makes 4 rolls

Chapter 5:

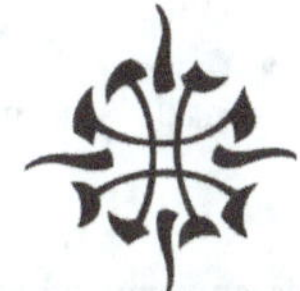

Avocado and Spinach Smoothie:

Ingredients:

- 1 ripe avocado, peeled and pitted

- 1 cup fresh spinach leaves

- 1 ripe banana

- 1 cup almond milk (or any other milk of your choice)

- 1 tablespoon honey or maple syrup (optional, for added sweetness)

- Juice of 1/2 lime (optional, for a tangy flavor)

- Ice cubes (optional, for a chilled smoothie)

Preparation:

1. In a blender, combine the avocado, spinach, banana, almond milk, honey or maple syrup (if using), and lime juice (if using).

2. Blend on high speed until smooth and creamy.

3. If desired, add a few ice cubes and blend again until the smoothie is chilled and frothy.

4. Taste the smoothie and adjust the sweetness or tanginess if needed by adding more honey, maple syrup, or lime juice.

5. Pour the avocado and spinach smoothie into glasses and serve immediately.

6. Enjoy the nutritious and creamy smoothie as a refreshing breakfast or snack.

Prep time: Approximately 5 minutes | Serves 2

Quinoa and Roasted Vegetable Salad:

Ingredients:

- 1 cup cooked quinoa

- 2 cups mixed roasted vegetables (such as bell peppers, zucchini, eggplant, and cherry tomatoes)

- 1/4 cup crumbled feta cheese

- 2 tablespoons chopped fresh herbs (such as parsley, basil, or cilantro)

- 2 tablespoons extra virgin olive oil

- 1 tablespoon lemon juice

- Salt and pepper to taste

Preparation:

1. In a large bowl, combine the cooked quinoa, roasted vegetables, crumbled feta cheese, and chopped fresh herbs.

2. In a small bowl, whisk together the olive oil, lemon juice, salt, and pepper to make the dressing.

3. Pour the dressing over the quinoa and roasted vegetable mixture and toss gently to coat all the ingredients.

4. Taste and adjust the seasoning if needed.

5. Serve the quinoa and roasted vegetable salad as a hearty and flavorful side dish or light lunch.

Prep time: Varies depending on quinoa cooking time and roasting vegetables | Serves 2-4

Ingredients:

- 2 salmon fillets

- 2 tablespoons melted butter or olive oil

- 2 cloves garlic, minced

- Zest of 1 lemon

- Juice of 1/2 lemon

- Salt and pepper to taste

- Fresh herbs (such as dill or parsley), chopped (optional, for garnish)

Preparation:

1. Preheat the oven to 375°F (190°C) and line a baking sheet with parchment paper.

2. Place the salmon fillets on the prepared baking sheet.

3. In a small bowl, mix together the melted butter or olive oil, minced garlic, lemon zest, lemon juice, salt, and pepper.

4. Pour the lemon garlic mixture over the salmon fillets, ensuring they are evenly coated.

5. Bake in the preheated oven for approximately 12-15 minutes, or until the salmon is cooked through and flakes easily with a fork.

6. Remove the salmon from the oven and let it rest for a few minutes.

7. Garnish with fresh herbs (if using) and serve the lemon garlic baked salmon with your choice of sides, such as roasted vegetables or quinoa.

Prep time: Approximately 10 minutes | Cook time: Approximately 12-15 minutes | Serves 2

Ingredients:

- 1 cup quinoa

- 1 can (13.5 ounces) coconut milk

- 1 cup vegetable broth or water

- 1 tablespoon curry powder

- 1/2 teaspoon turmeric powder

- 1/2 teaspoon cumin powder

- 1/2 teaspoon garlic powder

- 1/2 teaspoon salt

- Fresh cilantro, chopped (optional, for garnish)

Preparation:

1. Rinse the quinoa thoroughly under cold water.

2. In a saucepan, combine the rinsed quinoa, coconut milk, vegetable broth or water, curry powder, turmeric powder, cumin powder, garlic powder, and salt.

3. Bring the mixture to a boil over medium-high heat.

4. Reduce the heat to low, cover the saucepan, and simmer for about 15-20 minutes, or until the quinoa is cooked and the liquid is absorbed.

5. Remove the saucepan from the heat and let it sit, covered, for 5 minutes.

6. Fluff the quinoa with a fork and garnish with fresh chopped cilantro (if using).

7. Serve the coconut curry quinoa as a flavorful and aromatic side dish or as a base for a main course.

Prep time: Approximately 5 minutes | Cook time: Approximately 20 minutes | Serves 4

Ingredients:

- 1 cup dried lentils (green or brown), rinsed and drained

- 1 tablespoon vegetable oil

- 1 onion, finely chopped

- 2 cloves garlic, minced

- 1 tablespoon curry powder

- 1 teaspoon ground cumin

- 1 teaspoon ground coriander

- 1/2 teaspoon turmeric powder

- 1/4 teaspoon cayenne pepper (optional, for heat)

- 1 can (14 ounces) diced tomatoes

- 1 can (13.5 ounces) coconut milk

- 2 cups fresh spinach leaves

- Salt to taste

- Fresh cilantro, chopped (optional, for garnish)

- Cooked rice or naan bread, for serving

Preparation:

1. In a large saucepan, heat the vegetable oil over medium heat.

2. Add the chopped onion and minced garlic to the saucepan and sauté until the onion is soft and translucent.

3. Add the curry powder, cumin, coriander, turmeric, and cayenne pepper (if using) to the saucepan. Stir well to coat the onions and garlic with the spices.

4. Add the rinsed lentils, diced tomatoes (with their juices), and coconut milk to the saucepan. Stir to combine all the ingredients.

5. Bring the mixture to a boil, then reduce the heat to low, cover the saucepan, and simmer for about 20-25 minutes, or until the lentils are tender and cooked through.

6. Stir in the fresh spinach leaves and cook for an additional 2-3 minutes, or until the spinach wilts.

7. Taste the curry and season with salt according to your preference.

8. Serve the lentil and spinach curry over cooked rice or with naan bread. Garnish with fresh chopped cilantro (if using).

Prep time: Approximately 10 minutes | Cook time: Approximately 30 minutes | Serves 4-6

Ingredients:

- 1 cup Greek yogurt

- 1 cup mixed berries (such as strawberries, blueberries, raspberries)

- 1 ripe banana

- 1 tablespoon honey or maple syrup (optional, for added sweetness)

- 1/2 cup almond milk (or any other milk of your choice)

- Ice cubes (optional, for a chilled smoothie)

Preparation:

1. In a blender, combine the Greek yogurt, mixed berries, banana, honey or maple syrup (if using), and almond milk.

2. Blend on high speed until smooth and creamy.

3. If desired, add a few ice cubes and blend again until the smoothie is chilled and frothy.

4. Pour the Greek yogurt and berry smoothie into glasses and serve immediately.

5. Enjoy the refreshing and protein-packed smoothie as a nutritious breakfast or snack.

Prep time: Approximately 5 minutes | Serves 2

Ingredients:

- 1 pound shrimp, peeled and deveined

- 2 tablespoons olive oil

- 4 cloves garlic, minced

- 1 tablespoon chopped fresh herbs (such as parsley, basil, or dill)

- Juice of 1/2 lemon

- Salt and pepper to taste

Preparation:

1. Preheat the oven to 400°F (200°C) and line a baking sheet with parchment paper.

2. In a bowl, combine the shrimp, olive oil, minced garlic, fresh herbs, lemon juice, salt, and pepper. Toss to coat the shrimp evenly.

3. Arrange the seasoned shrimp in a single layer on the prepared baking sheet.

4. Roast in the preheated oven for approximately 8-10 minutes, or until the shrimp are pink and cooked through.

5. Remove the shrimp from the oven and let them rest for a few minutes.

6. Serve the garlic herb roasted shrimp as an appetizer, main course with pasta or rice, or as a protein topping for salads.

Prep time: Approximately 10 minutes | Cook time: Approximately 8-10 minutes | Serves 2-4

Stuffed Bell Peppers with Quinoa and Feta:

Ingredients:

- 4 bell peppers (any color), tops removed and seeds discarded

- 1 cup cooked quinoa

- 1/2 cup crumbled feta cheese

- 1/4 cup chopped sun-dried tomatoes

- 1/4 cup chopped fresh herbs (such as parsley or basil)

- 2 tablespoons olive oil

- 2 cloves garlic, minced

- Salt and pepper to taste

Preparation:

1. Preheat the oven to 375°F (190°C) and lightly grease a baking dish.

2. In a bowl, combine the cooked quinoa, crumbled feta cheese, chopped sun-dried tomatoes, chopped fresh herbs, olive oil, minced garlic, salt, and pepper. Mix well.

3. Stuff the bell peppers with the quinoa and feta mixture, pressing it down gently to fill the peppers completely.

4. Place the stuffed bell peppers in the prepared baking dish.

5. Bake in the preheated oven for approximately 25-30 minutes, or until the peppers are tender and the filling is heated through.

6. Remove the stuffed bell peppers from the oven and let them cool for a few minutes before serving.

7. Serve the stuffed bell peppers with quinoa and feta as a satisfying and flavorful vegetarian main dish.

Prep time: Approximately 15 minutes | Cook time: Approximately 25-30 minutes | Serves 4

Ingredients:

- 1 cup rolled oats

- 1/2 cup almond butter

- 1/4 cup honey or maple syrup

- 1/4 cup chopped nuts (such as almonds or walnuts)

- 1/4 cup dried fruits (such as raisins or cranberries)

- 1 tablespoon chia seeds

- 1 teaspoon vanilla extract

- Pinch of salt

- Desiccated coconut or cocoa powder (for coating, optional)

Preparation:

1. In a large bowl, combine the rolled oats, almond butter, honey or maple syrup, chopped nuts, dried fruits, chia seeds, vanilla extract, and salt. Mix well until all the ingredients are evenly combined.

2. Form the mixture into small bite-sized balls using your hands. If desired, roll the energy balls in desiccated coconut or cocoa powder for an extra layer of flavor and texture.

3. Place the energy balls on a baking sheet or a plate and refrigerate for at least 1 hour to firm up.

4. Once chilled, the almond butter energy balls are ready to be enjoyed. Store any leftovers in an airtight container in the refrigerator for up to one week.

Prep time: Approximately 15 minutes | Chill time: At least 1 hour | Makes about 15 energy balls

Ingredients:

- Assorted vegetables of your choice (such as carrots, cauliflower, Brussels sprouts, sweet potatoes, and zucchini), cut into bite-sized pieces

- 2 tablespoons olive oil

- 1 teaspoon ground turmeric

- 1/2 teaspoon ground cumin

- 1/2 teaspoon ground paprika

- 1/2 teaspoon salt

- 1/4 teaspoon black pepper

- Fresh cilantro or parsley for garnish (optional)

Preparation:

1. Preheat the oven to 400°F (200°C) and line a baking sheet with parchment paper.

2. In a large bowl, combine the olive oil, ground turmeric, ground cumin, ground paprika, salt, and black pepper. Stir well to make a spice mixture.

3. Add the bite-sized vegetables to the bowl and toss them with the spice mixture until evenly coated.

4. Spread the seasoned vegetables in a single layer on the prepared baking sheet.

5. Roast in the preheated oven for approximately 25-30 minutes, or until the vegetables are tender and golden brown, stirring once halfway through.

6. Remove the roasted vegetables from the oven and let them cool slightly.

7. Garnish with fresh cilantro or parsley, if desired, and serve as a flavorful side dish or as a base for grain bowls or salads.

Prep time: Approximately 15 minutes | Cook time: Approximately 25-30 minutes | Serves 4-6

Mediterranean Pasta Salad:

Ingredients:

- 8 ounces (225g) pasta of your choice (such as penne or fusilli)

- 1 cup cherry tomatoes, halved

- 1 cucumber, diced

- 1/2 red onion, thinly sliced

- 1/2 cup Kalamata olives, pitted and halved

- 1/2 cup crumbled feta cheese

- 1/4 cup chopped fresh parsley

- 2 tablespoons extra virgin olive oil

- 2 tablespoons red wine vinegar

- 1 clove garlic, minced

- 1 teaspoon dried oregano

- Salt and pepper to taste

Preparation:

1. Cook the pasta according to the package instructions until al dente. Drain and rinse with cold water to stop the cooking process.

2. In a large bowl, combine the cooked pasta, cherry tomatoes, cucumber, red onion, Kalamata olives, feta cheese, and chopped parsley.

3. In a small bowl, whisk together the olive oil, red wine vinegar, minced garlic, dried oregano, salt, and pepper to make the dressing.

4. Pour the dressing over the pasta salad and toss gently to coat all the ingredients.

5. Cover the bowl and refrigerate for at least 1 hour to allow the flavors to meld.

6. Before serving, give the Mediterranean pasta salad a quick toss to redistribute the dressing. Adjust the seasoning if needed.

7. Serve the pasta salad chilled as a refreshing side dish or light meal.

Prep time: Approximately 15 minutes | Cook time: Varies based on pasta type | Chill time: At least 1 hour | Serves 4-6

Ingredients:

- 1 cup cooked quinoa

- 12 ounces (340g) canned or cooked salmon, drained and flaked

- 1/4 cup breadcrumbs

- 1/4 cup chopped fresh herbs (such as dill, parsley, or cilantro)

- 2 green onions, finely chopped

- 1 clove garlic, minced

- 1 tablespoon lemon juice

- 2 eggs, lightly beaten

- Salt and pepper to taste

- 2 tablespoons olive oil (for cooking)

Preparation:

1. In a large bowl, combine the cooked quinoa, flaked salmon, breadcrumbs, chopped fresh herbs, green onions, minced garlic, lemon juice, beaten eggs, salt, and pepper. Mix well until all the ingredients are evenly incorporated.

2. Shape the mixture into patties of your desired size, compacting them gently to hold their shape.

3. Heat the olive oil in a skillet over medium heat.

4. Cook the salmon and quinoa patties in the skillet for approximately 3-4 minutes per side, or until golden brown and cooked through.

5. Once cooked, transfer the patties to a plate lined with paper towels to absorb any excess oil.

6. Serve the salmon and quinoa patties as a protein-rich main dish, either on their own or in a burger bun with your favorite toppings.

Prep time: Approximately 15 minutes | Cook time: Approximately 8-10 minutes | Makes 4-6 patties

Berry Spinach Smoothie:

Ingredients:

- 1 cup fresh or frozen mixed berries (such as strawberries, blueberries, raspberries)

- 1 ripe banana

- 2 cups fresh spinach leaves

- 1 cup almond milk (or any other milk of your choice)

- 1 tablespoon honey or maple syrup (optional, for added sweetness)

- Ice cubes (optional, for a chilled smoothie)

Preparation:

1. In a blender, combine the mixed berries, ripe banana, fresh spinach leaves, almond milk, and honey or maple syrup (if using).

2. Blend on high speed until smooth and creamy.

3. If desired, add a few ice cubes and blend again until the smoothie is chilled and frothy.

4. Pour the berry spinach smoothie into glasses and serve immediately.

5. Enjoy this nutrient-packed smoothie as a refreshing breakfast or snack.

Prep time: Approximately 5 minutes | Serves 2

Ingredients:

- 2 boneless, skinless chicken breasts

- 4 slices mozzarella cheese

- 2 large tomato slices

- 4 fresh basil leaves

- 2 tablespoons balsamic glaze

- Salt and pepper to taste

- Olive oil for cooking

Preparation:

1. Preheat the oven to 400°F (200°C).

2. Butterfly the chicken breasts by slicing them horizontally, but not all the way through, so you can open them like a book.

3. Season the inside of the chicken breasts with salt and pepper.

4. Place 2 slices of mozzarella cheese, 1 tomato slice, and 2 basil leaves inside each chicken breast. Close the chicken breasts to enclose the filling.

55. Use toothpicks to secure the chicken breasts, if needed.

6. Heat some olive oil in an oven-safe skillet over medium-high heat.

7. Sear the stuffed chicken breasts for about 2-3 minutes on each side until golden brown.

8. Transfer the skillet to the preheated oven and bake for approximately 15-20 minutes, or until the chicken is cooked through and the cheese is melted and bubbly.

9. Remove the skillet from the oven and let the chicken rest for a few minutes.

10. Drizzle the chicken breasts with balsamic glaze before serving.

11. Serve the caprese stuffed chicken breast as a delicious and flavorful main dish with a side of vegetables or salad.

Prep time: Approximately 15 minutes | Cook time: Approximately 25-30 minutes | Serves 2

Ingredients:

- 1 can (15 ounces) chickpeas, drained and rinsed

- 1/2 cup roasted red peppers (from a jar), drained

- 2 tablespoons tahini

- 2 tablespoons lemon juice

- 1 clove garlic, minced

- 2 tablespoons olive oil

- 1/2 teaspoon ground cumin

- Salt and pepper to taste

- Optional toppings: olive oil, paprika, chopped fresh parsley

Preparation:

1. In a food processor or blender, combine the chickpeas, roasted red peppers, tahini, lemon juice, minced garlic, olive oil, ground cumin, salt, and pepper.

2. Process or blend until smooth and creamy, scraping down the sides as needed.

3. Taste the hummus and adjust the seasoning if needed by adding more salt, pepper, or lemon juice.

4. Transfer the hummus to a serving bowl.

5. If desired, drizzle some olive oil over the top and sprinkle with paprika and chopped fresh parsley for garnish.

6. Serve the roasted red pepper hummus with pita bread, crackers, or fresh vegetables for dipping.

Prep time: Approximately 10 minutes | Makes about 1 1/2 cups of hummus

Quinoa and Black Bean Quesadillas:

Ingredients:

- 1 cup cooked quinoa

- 1 cup canned black beans, rinsed and drained

- 1 cup shredded cheese (such as cheddar or Monterey Jack)

- 1/2 cup diced bell peppers (any color)

- 1/4 cup chopped fresh cilantro

- 1/2 teaspoon ground cumin

- 1/2 teaspoon chili powder

- Salt and pepper to taste

- 4 large flour tortillas

- Olive oil for cooking

- Optional toppings: salsa, sour cream, guacamole

Preparation:

1. In a large bowl, combine the cooked quinoa, black beans, shredded cheese, diced bell peppers, chopped cilantro, ground cumin, chili powder,

salt, and pepper. Mix well to ensure all the ingredients are evenly distributed.

2. Heat a lightly oiled skillet or griddle over medium heat.

3. Place a tortilla on the skillet and spoon a quarter of the quinoa and black bean mixture onto one half of the tortilla.

4. Fold the other half of the tortilla over the filling to create a quesadilla. Press down gently.

5. Cook the quesadilla for approximately 2-3 minutes on each side, or until golden brown and the cheese is melted.

6. Repeat the process with the remaining tortillas and filling.

7. Once cooked, remove the quesadillas from the skillet and cut them into wedges.

8. Serve the quinoa and black bean quesadillas warm with salsa, sour cream, and guacamole as desired.

Prep time: Approximately 10 minutes | Cook time: Approximately 10 minutes | Makes 4 quesadillas

Lemon Poppy Seed Overnight Oats:

Ingredients:

- 1/2 cup rolled oats

- 1/2 cup milk (dairy or plant-based)

- 1/2 cup Greek yogurt

- 1 tablespoon honey or maple syrup

- 1 tablespoon fresh lemon juice

- 1/2 teaspoon lemon zest

- 1 teaspoon poppy seeds

- Optional toppings: fresh berries, sliced almonds, additional honey or maple syrup

Preparation:

1. In a jar or container with a lid, combine the rolled oats, milk, Greek yogurt, honey or maple syrup, lemon juice, lemon zest, and poppy seeds.

2. Stir well to ensure all the ingredients are evenly mixed.

3. Cover the jar or container and refrigerate overnight, or for at least 4 hours, to allow the oats to soak and soften.

4. In the morning, give the overnight oats a good stir.

5. If desired, top the oats with fresh berries, sliced almonds, and a drizzle of honey or maple syrup.

6. Enjoy the lemon poppy seed overnight oats cold or at room temperature for a quick and nutritious breakfast.

Prep time: Approximately 5 minutes (plus chilling time) | Serves 1

Baked Sweet Potato Fries:

Ingredients:

- 2 large sweet potatoes

- 2 tablespoons olive oil

- 1 teaspoon paprika

- 1/2 teaspoon garlic powder

- 1/2 teaspoon salt

- 1/4 teaspoon black pepper

Preparation:

1. Preheat the oven to 425°F (220°C).

2. Peel the sweet potatoes and cut them into thin fries or wedges.

3. In a large bowl, combine the sweet potato fries, olive oil, paprika, garlic powder, salt, and black pepper. Toss well to coat the fries evenly with the seasonings.

4. Spread the seasoned sweet potato fries in a single layer on a baking sheet lined with parchment paper.

5. Bake in the preheated oven for approximately 20-25 minutes, flipping the fries halfway through, until they are golden brown and crispy.

6. Once baked, remove the sweet potato fries from the oven and let them cool for a few minutes before serving.

7. Serve the baked sweet potato fries as a healthier alternative to traditional french fries, with your favorite dipping sauce.

Prep time: Approximately 10 minutes | Cook time: Approximately 20-25 minutes | Serves 2-4

Ingredients:

- 3 large eggs

- 1 tablespoon milk

- 1/2 cup fresh spinach leaves

- 1/4 cup sliced mushrooms

- 1/4 cup shredded cheese (such as cheddar or Swiss)

- 1 tablespoon butter or olive oil

- Salt and pepper to taste

Preparation:

1. In a bowl, whisk together the eggs and milk. Season with salt and pepper.

2. Heat the butter or olive oil in a non-stick skillet over medium heat.

3. Add the spinach leaves and sliced mushrooms to the skillet. Sauté for a few minutes until the spinach wilts and the mushrooms soften.

4. Pour the whisked eggs overthe sautéed spinach and mushrooms in the skillet.

5. Allow the eggs to cook undisturbed for a minute or two until the edges start to set.

6. Gently lift the edges of the omelette with a spatula and tilt the skillet to allow the uncooked eggs to flow to the edges.

7. Sprinkle the shredded cheese evenly over one half of the omelette.

8. Using the spatula, carefully fold the other half of the omelette over the cheese to create a half-moon shape.

9. Cook for another minute or until the cheese melts and the omelette is cooked to your desired level of doneness.

10. Slide the spinach and mushroom omelette onto a plate and serve hot.

Prep time: Approximately 5 minutes | Cook time: Approximately 5 minutes | Serves 1

Avocado and Tomato Bruschetta:

Ingredients:

- 1 baguette, sliced into 1/2-inch thick slices

- 2 ripe avocados

- 1 cup cherry tomatoes, halved

- 1/4 cup chopped fresh basil

- 1 tablespoon lemon juice

- 1 clove garlic, minced

- 2 tablespoons extra virgin olive oil

- Salt and pepper to taste

Preparation:

1. Preheat the oven to 375°F (190°C).

2. Place the baguette slices on a baking sheet and brush both sides with olive oil.

3. Bake the baguette slices in the preheated oven for about 10 minutes, or until they are golden and crispy.

4. While the baguette slices are toasting, prepare the avocado and tomato topping.

5. In a bowl, mash the ripe avocados with a fork until they reach your desired consistency.

6. Add the halved cherry tomatoes, chopped fresh basil, lemon juice, minced garlic, and extra virgin olive oil to the mashed avocados. Mix well to combine.

7. Season the avocado and tomato mixture with salt and pepper to taste.

8. Once the baguette slices are done, remove them from the oven and let them cool slightly.

9. Spoon the avocado and tomato mixture onto the toasted baguette slices, distributing it evenly.

10. Serve the avocado and tomato bruschetta as an appetizer or a light snack.

Prep time: Approximately 10 minutes | Cook time: Approximately 10 minutes | Serves 4-6

Chapter 6:

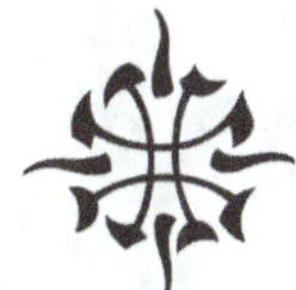

BRAIN-BOOSTING DESSERTS

Dark Chocolate and Berry Smoothie:

Ingredients:

- 1 cup frozen mixed berries (such as strawberries, blueberries, and raspberries)

- 1 ripe banana

- 1 tablespoon unsweetened cocoa powder

- 1 tablespoon honey or maple syrup (optional, for added sweetness)

- 1 cup milk (dairy or plant-based)

- 1/2 cup Greek yogurt (optional, for added creaminess)

- Ice cubes (optional, for a colder smoothie)

Instructions:

1. Place the frozen mixed berries, ripe banana, unsweetened cocoa powder, honey or maple syrup (if using), milk, and Greek yogurt (if using) in a blender.

2. Blend on high speed until all the ingredients are well combined and the smoothie is creamy and smooth.

3. If desired, add a few ice cubes and blend again to make the smoothie colder.

4. Taste the smoothie and adjust the sweetness by adding more honey or maple syrup if desired.

5. Pour the dark chocolate and berry smoothie into glasses and serve immediately.

Ingredients:

- 1/4 cup chia seeds

- 1 cup coconut milk (canned or homemade)

- 1 tablespoon honey or maple syrup (optional, for added sweetness)

- 1/2 teaspoon vanilla extract

- Fresh fruits or berries for topping

Instructions:

1. In a bowl, combine the chia seeds, coconut milk, honey or maple syrup (if using), and vanilla extract.

2. Whisk the mixture well to ensure the chia seeds are evenly distributed and not clumping together.

3. Let the mixture sit for about 5 minutes, then give it another good stir.

4. Cover the bowl and refrigerate the chia seed and coconut mixture for at least 2 hours, or overnight, until it thickens and develops a pudding-like consistency.

5. Once the pudding has set, give it a final stir to break up any clumps.

6. Serve the chia seed and coconut pudding in individual bowls or jars, and top with fresh fruits or berries of your choice.

7. Enjoy the pudding chilled as a healthy and delicious dessert or breakfast option.

Ingredients:

- 1 3/4 cups all-purpose flour

- 1/2 cup granulated sugar

- 2 teaspoons baking powder

- 1/4 teaspoon salt

- 1 tablespoon chia seeds

- 1 cup milk (dairy or plant-based)

- 1/4 cup vegetable oil

- 1 teaspoon vanilla extract

- Zest and juice of 1 lemon

- 1 cup fresh or frozen blueberries

Instructions:

1. Preheat the oven to 375°F (190°C) and line a muffin tin with paper liners or grease the cups.

2. In a large bowl, whisk together the all-purpose flour, granulated sugar, baking powder, salt, and chia seeds.

3. In a separate bowl, combine the milk, vegetable oil, vanilla extract, lemon zest, and lemon juice.

4. Pour the wet ingredients into the dry ingredients and stir until just combined. Do not overmix.

5. Gently fold in the blueberries.

6. Spoon the batter into the prepared muffin cups, filling each cup about 2/3 full.

7. Bake in the preheated oven for approximately 18-20 minutes, or until a toothpick inserted into the center of a muffin comes out clean.

8. Remove the muffins from the oven and let them cool in the tin for a few minutes before transferring them to a wire rack to cool completely.

9. Serve the lemon blueberry chia seed muffins as a delightful breakfast or snack option.

Ingredients:

- 1 cup pitted dates

- 1 cup unsweetened shredded coconut

- Zest and juice of 1 lime

- 1/4 cup raw almonds

- 1 tablespoon chia seeds

- 1 tablespoon honey or maple syrup (optional, for added sweetness)

- Extra shredded coconut for rolling (optional)

Instructions:

1. Place the pitted dates, unsweetened shredded coconut, lime zest and juice, raw almonds, chia seeds, and honey or maple syrup (if using) in a food processor.

2. Process the ingredients until they are well combined and form a sticky mixture.

3. Scoop out tablespoon-sized portions of the mixture and roll them into balls using your hands.

4. If desired, roll the energy bites in extra shredded coconut to coat them.

5. Place the coconut lime energy bites in an airtight container and refrigerate them for at least 1 hour to firm up.

6. Once chilled, the energy bites are ready to be enjoyed as a healthy snack or on-the-go energy boost.

Chocolate Avocado Mousse

Ingredients:

- 2 ripe avocados

- 1/3 cup cocoa powder

- 1/4 cup honey or maple syrup

- 1/4 cup milk (dairy or plant-based)

- 1 teaspoon vanilla extract

- Pinch of salt

- Optional toppings: whipped cream, shaved chocolate, berries

Instructions:

1. Cut the avocados in half, remove the pits, and scoop out the flesh into a blender or food processor.

2. Add the cocoa powder, honey or maple syrup, milk, vanilla extract, and salt to the blender or food processor.

3. Blend the ingredients until smooth and creamy, scraping down the sides as needed.

4. Taste the mousse and adjust the sweetness by adding more honey or maple syrup if desired.

5. Spoon the chocolate avocado mousse into serving bowls or glasses.

6. If desired, top the mousse with whipped cream, shaved chocolate, or fresh berries.

7. Refrigerate the mousse for at least 30 minutes to chill and set.

8. Serve the chocolate avocado mousse chilled as a decadent and healthier dessert option.

Ingredients:

- 1 cup Greek yogurt

- 1 cup mixed berries (such as strawberries, blueberries, and raspberries)

- 2 tablespoons honey or maple syrup

- Popsicle molds

- Popsicle sticks

Instructions:

1. In a blender, combine the Greek yogurt, mixed berries, and honey or maple syrup.

2. Blend until smooth and well combined.

3. Pour the mixture into popsicle molds, filling each mold about 3/4 full.

4. Insert popsicle sticks into the molds.

5. Place the molds in the freezer and freeze for at least 4-6 hours, or until the popsicles are completely frozen.

6. Once frozen, remove the popsicles from the molds and enjoy these refreshing Greek yogurt and berry popsicles.

Ingredients:

- 1 cup almond flour

- 1/2 teaspoon baking powder

- 1/4 teaspoon salt

- 2 tablespoons honey or maple syrup

- 2 large eggs

- 1/4 cup milk (dairy or plant-based)

- 1 teaspoon vanilla extract

- 1/2 cup fresh blueberries

- Butter or oil for greasing the pan

Instructions:

1. In a bowl, whisk together the almond flour, baking powder, and salt.

2. In a separate bowl, whisk together the honey or maple syrup, eggs, milk, and vanilla extract.

3. Pour the wet ingredients into the dry ingredients and stir until well combined.

4. Gently fold in the fresh blueberries.

5. Heat a non-stick skillet or griddle over medium heat and grease it with butter or oil.

6. Spoon about 1/4 cup of batter onto the skillet for each pancake.

7. Cook the pancakes for 2-3 minutes on one side, until bubbles form on the surface.

8. Flip the pancakes and cook for an additional 1-2 minutes, or until golden brown.

9. Repeat with the remaining batter.

10. Serve the almond flour blueberry pancakes warm, topped with additional blueberries and your choice of syrup or honey.

Raspberry and Dark Chocolate Bark:

Ingredients:

- 8 ounces dark chocolate, chopped

- 1/2 cup fresh raspberries

- 2 tablespoons chopped almonds or other nuts (optional)

Instructions:

1. Line a baking sheet with parchment paper.

2. Melt the dark chocolate in a microwave-safe bowl in 30-second intervals, stirring in between, until completely melted and smooth.

3. Pour the melted chocolate onto the prepared baking sheet and spread it out evenly using a spatula.

4. Sprinkle the fresh raspberries and chopped almonds (if using) over the melted chocolate, pressing them gently into the chocolate.

5. Place the baking sheet in the refrigerator and chill for at least 1 hour, or until the chocolate has hardened.

6. Once hardened, break the raspberry and dark chocolate bark into smaller pieces.

7. Store the bark in an airtight container in the refrigerator.

8. Enjoy the sweet and tangy flavors of this delightful treat.

Lemon Poppy Seed Energy Balls:

Ingredients:

- 1 cup Medjool dates, pitted

- 1 cup raw cashews

- Zest and juice of 1 lemon

- 2 tablespoons poppy seeds

- 1/4 teaspoon vanilla extract

- Pinch of salt

- Unsweetened shredded coconut (optional, for rolling)

Instructions:

1. Place the Medjool dates, raw cashews, lemon zest and juice, poppy seeds, vanilla extract, and salt in a food processor.

2. Process the ingredients until they form a sticky mixture that holds together when pressed between your fingers.

3. Scoop out tablespoon-sized portions of the mixture and roll them into balls using your hands.

4. If desired, roll the energy balls in unsweetened shredded coconut to coat them.

5. Place the lemon poppy seed energy balls in an airtight container and refrigerate them for at least 1 hour to firm up.

6. Once chilled, the energy balls are ready to be enjoyed as a healthy and energizing snack.

Blackberry Coconut Chia Seed Parfait:

Ingredients:

- 1/2 cup blackberries

- 1/2 cup coconut yogurt (dairy or plant-based)

- 2 tablespoons chia seeds

- 1/4 cup granola

- Fresh mint leaves for garnish (optional)

Instructions:

1. In a bowl or glass, layer half of the blackberries at the bottom.

2. In a separate bowl, mix together the coconut yogurt and chia seeds until well combined. Let it sit for a few minutes to allow the chia seeds to absorb some liquid and thicken the mixture.

3. Spoon half of the chia seed mixture over the blackberries in the bowl orglass.

4. Add another layer of blackberries on top of the chia seed mixture.

5. Repeat the layers with the remaining blackberries and chia seed mixture.

6. Sprinkle granola on the top layer.

7. Garnish with fresh mint leaves if desired.

8. Serve the blackberry coconut chia seed parfait immediately or refrigerate for a few hours to allow the flavors to meld together.

9. Enjoy this delicious and nutritious parfait as a breakfast or snack option.

Ingredients:

- Fresh strawberries

- 8 ounces dark chocolate, chopped

- Optional toppings: chopped nuts, shredded coconut, sprinkles

Instructions:

1. Wash and dry the strawberries, leaving the stems intact.

2. Line a baking sheet with parchment paper.

3. Melt the dark chocolate in a microwave-safe bowl in 30-second intervals, stirring in between, until completely melted and smooth.

4. Hold a strawberry by the stem and dip it into the melted chocolate, allowing any excess chocolate to drip off.

5. If desired, roll the chocolate-covered strawberry in chopped nuts, shredded coconut, or sprinkles.

6. Place the chocolate-covered strawberry on the prepared baking sheet.

7. Repeat with the remaining strawberries.

8. Once all strawberries are coated, place the baking sheet in the refrigerator for about 15-20 minutes, or until the chocolate has hardened.

9. Serve the chocolate-covered strawberries as a delightful treat or as a romantic dessert.

Ingredients:

- 4 cups mixed berries (such as strawberries, blueberries, raspberries, and blackberries)

- 1/4 cup granulated sugar

- 1 tablespoon cornstarch

- 1 cup rolled oats

- 1/2 cup almond flour

- 1/4 cup honey or maple syrup

- 1/4 cup melted butter or coconut oil

- 1/2 teaspoon vanilla extract

- Pinch of salt

- Vanilla ice cream or whipped cream for serving (optional)

Instructions:

1. Preheat your oven to 350°F (175°C).

2. In a large bowl, combine the mixed berries, granulated sugar, and cornstarch. Toss gently to coat the berries evenly.

3. Transfer the berry mixture to a baking dish or individual ramekins.

4. In another bowl, mix together the rolled oats, almond flour, honey or maple syrup, melted butter or coconut oil, vanilla extract, and salt until well combined.

5. Sprinkle the oat mixture evenly over the berries in the baking dish.

6. Bake in the preheated oven for 25-30 minutes, or until the berries are bubbling and the crumble topping is golden brown.

7. Remove from the oven and let it cool for a few minutes.

8. Serve the mixed berry crumble warm, with a scoop of vanilla ice cream or a dollop of whipped cream, if desired.

Ingredients:

- 1 cup all-purpose flour

- 1/2 cup granulated sugar

- 1/2 teaspoon baking powder

- 1/4 teaspoon salt

- 2 large eggs

- 1/2 teaspoon vanilla extract

- 1/2 cup shelled pistachios, coarsely chopped

- 1/2 cup dark chocolate chips or chopped dark chocolate

Instructions:

1. Preheat your oven to 350°F (175°C) and line a baking sheet with parchment paper.

2. In a bowl, whisk together the flour, granulated sugar, baking powder, and salt.

3. In a separate bowl, beat the eggs and vanilla extract together.

4. Add the egg mixture to the flour mixture and stir until a dough forms.

5. Fold in the pistachios and dark chocolate chips or chopped dark chocolate.

6. Transfer the dough to the prepared baking sheet and shape it into a log, about 12 inches long and 3 inches wide.

7. Bake in the preheated oven for 25-30 minutes, or until the log is firm to the touch and lightly golden brown.

8. Remove the log from the oven and let it cool on the baking sheet for 10 minutes.

9. Using a sharp knife, slice the log diagonally into 1/2-inch thick biscotti.

10. Place the biscotti back on the baking sheet, cut side down.

11. Reduce the oven temperature to 325°F (165°C) and bake the biscotti for an additional 10-15 minutes, or until they are crisp and golden.

12. Remove from the oven and let the biscotti cool completely before serving.

13. Enjoy these crunchy pistachio and dark chocolate biscotti with a cup of coffee or tea.

Ingredients:

- 1 1/2 cups almond flour

- 1/4 cup melted coconut oil or butter

- 2 tablespoons honey or maple syrup

- 1 cup Greek yogurt

- 2 tablespoons honey or maple syrup

- 1 teaspoon vanilla extract

- Assorted fresh berries for topping

Instructions:

1. Preheat your oven to 350°F (175°C).

2. In a bowl, combine the almond flour, melted coconut oil or butter, and honey or maple syrup. Mix until well combined and the mixture resembles coarse crumbs.

3. Press the almond flourmixture into the bottom of a tart pan, spreading it evenly to form the crust.

4. Bake the crust in the preheated oven for 10-12 minutes, or until it is golden brown. Remove from the oven and let it cool completely.

5. In a separate bowl, whisk together the Greek yogurt, honey or maple syrup, and vanilla extract until smooth.

6. Once the crust has cooled, spread the Greek yogurt mixture evenly over the crust.

7. Arrange the fresh berries on top of the Greek yogurt mixture.

8. Refrigerate the tart for at least 1 hour before serving to allow the flavors to meld together and the tart to set.

9. Slice and serve the Greek yogurt and berry tart as a refreshing and delicious dessert.

Ingredients:

- 2 cups almond flour

- 1/2 teaspoon baking soda

- 1/4 teaspoon salt

- 1/4 cup melted coconut oil or butter

- 1/4 cup honey or maple syrup

- 1 teaspoon vanilla extract

- 1/2 cup dark chocolate chips

Instructions:

1. Preheat your oven to 350°F (175°C) and line a baking sheet with parchment paper.

2. In a bowl, whisk together the almond flour, baking soda, and salt.

3. In a separate bowl, mix together the melted coconut oil or butter, honey or maple syrup, and vanilla extract.

4. Add the wet ingredients to the dry ingredients and stir until well combined.

5. Fold in the dark chocolate chips.

6. Drop tablespoon-sized portions of dough onto the prepared baking sheet, spacing them a few inches apart.

7. Flatten each cookie slightly with the back of a spoon or your fingers.

8. Bake in the preheated oven for 10-12 minutes, or until the cookies are golden brown around the edges.

9. Remove from the oven and let the cookies cool on the baking sheet for a few minutes before transferring them to a wire rack to cool completely.

10. Enjoy these almond flour chocolate chip cookies as a healthier alternative to traditional cookies.

Ingredients:

- 1 3/4 cups all-purpose flour

- 1 1/2 teaspoons baking powder

- 1/4 teaspoon salt

- 1 tablespoon poppy seeds

- 1 cup unsalted butter, softened

- 1 1/2 cups granulated sugar

- 4 large eggs

- 2 teaspoons lemon zest

- 1/4 cup fresh lemon juice

- 1/2 cup milk

- 1 teaspoon vanilla extract

Instructions:

1. Preheat your oven to 350°F (175°C) and grease a loaf pan.

2. In a bowl, whisk together the flour, baking powder, salt, and poppy seeds.

3. In a separate bowl, cream together the softened butter and granulated sugar until light and fluffy.

4. Beat in the eggs, one at a time, mixing well after each addition.

5. Stir in the lemon zest, lemon juice, milk, and vanilla extract.

6. Gradually add the dry ingredients to the wet ingredients, mixing until just combined.

7. Pour the batter into the greased loaf pan and smooth the top.

8. Bake in the preheated oven for 50-60 minutes, or until a toothpick inserted into the center comes out clean.

9. Remove from the oven and let the pound cake cool in the pan for 10 minutes.

10. Transfer the cake to a wire rack to cool completely before slicing and serving.

Ingredients:

- 3 cups ripe mango chunks (fresh or frozen)

- 1 cup coconut milk

- 1/4 cup honey or maple syrup

- 1 tablespoon lime juice

- Shredded coconut for garnish (optional)

Instructions:

1. Place the mango chunks, coconut milk, honey or maple syrup, and lime juice in a blender or food processor.

2. Blend until smooth and creamy.

3. Pour the mixture into an ice cream maker and churn according to the manufacturer's instructions until it reaches a sorbet-like consistency.

4. If you don't have an ice cream maker, pour the mixture into a shallow dish and place it in the freezer. Every 30 minutes, remove the dish from the freezer and use a fork to stir and break up any ice crystals. Repeat this process until the sorbet is firm and scoopable.

5. Once the sorbet reaches the desired consistency, transfer it to a lidded container and freeze for an additional 1-2 hours to firm up.

6. Serve the coconut mango sorbet in bowls or cones, garnished with shredded coconut if desired.

Dark Chocolate and Walnut Brownies:

Ingredients:

- 1 cup unsalted butter

- 2 cups granulated sugar

- 4 large eggs

- 1 teaspoon vanilla extract

- 1 cup all-purpose flour

- 1/2 cup unsweetened cocoa powder

- 1/4 teaspoon salt

- 1 cup dark chocolate chips

- 1 cup chopped walnuts

Instructions:

1. Preheat your oven to 350°F (175°C) and grease a baking dish.

2. In a microwave-safe bowl, melt the butter.

3. In a separate bowl, whisk together the melted butter and granulated sugar.

4. Beat in the eggs, one at a time, mixing well after each addition.

5. Stir in the vanilla extract.

6. In another bowl, sift together the flour, cocoa powder, and salt.

7. Gradually add the dry ingredients to the wet ingredients, mixing until just combined.

8. Fold in the dark chocolate chips and chopped walnuts.

9. Pour the batter into the greased baking dish and spread it evenly.

10. Bake in the preheated oven for 25-30 minutes, or until a toothpick inserted into the center comes out with a few moist crumbs.

11. Remove from the oven and let the brownies cool completely in the baking dish before cutting into squares.

Mixed Berry Frozen Yogurt:

Ingredients:

- 3 cups mixed berries (such as strawberries, blueberries, raspberries, and blackberries), fresh or frozen

- 2 cups plain Greek yogurt

- 1/2 cup honey or maple syrup

- 1 tablespoon fresh lemon juice

Instructions:

1. Place the mixed berries, Greek yogurt, honey or maple syrup, and lemon juice in a blender or food processor.

2. Blend until smooth and well combined.

3. Taste the mixture and adjust the sweetness with additional honey or maple syrup if needed.

4. Pour the mixture into an ice cream maker and churn according to the manufacturer's instructions until it reaches a frozen yogurt consistency.

5. If you don't have an ice cream maker, pour the mixture into a shallow dish and place it in the freezer. Every 30 minutes, remove the dish from the freezer and use a fork to stir and break upany ice crystals. Repeat this process until the frozen yogurt is creamy and scoopable.

6. Once the desired consistency is reached, transfer the frozen yogurt to a lidded container and freeze for an additional 1-2 hours to firm up.

7. Serve the mixed berry frozen yogurt in bowls or cones.

Ingredients:

For the crust:

- 1 1/2 cups graham cracker crumbs

- 1/4 cup granulated sugar

- 1/2 cup unsalted butter, melted

For the cheesecake filling:

- 16 ounces cream cheese, softened

- 1/2 cup granulated sugar

- 2 large eggs

- 1 tablespoon lemon zest

- 1 tablespoon fresh lemon juice

- 1 teaspoon vanilla extract

For the raspberry swirl:

- 1/2 cup raspberry preserves or jam

Instructions:

1. Preheat your oven to 325°F (160°C) and line a baking dish with parchment paper, leaving an overhang on the sides for easy removal.

2. In a bowl, combine the graham cracker crumbs, granulated sugar, and melted butter for the crust. Mix until the crumbs are evenly coated.

3. Press the crust mixture into the bottom of the prepared baking dish in an even layer.

4. In a separate bowl, beat the cream cheese and granulated sugar together until smooth and creamy.

5. Add the eggs, one at a time, beating well after each addition.

6. Stir in the lemon zest, lemon juice, and vanilla extract.

7. Pour the cheesecake filling over the crust in the baking dish, spreading it out evenly.

8. Drop spoonfuls of raspberry preserves or jam onto the cheesecake filling.

9. Use a knife or toothpick to swirl the raspberry preserves into the cheesecake filling, creating a marbled effect.

10. Bake in the preheated oven for 40-45 minutes, or until the edges are set and the center is slightly jiggly.

11. Remove from the oven and let the cheesecake bars cool completely in the baking dish.

12. Once cooled, refrigerate for at least 3 hours or overnight to allow the bars to firm up.

13. Lift the bars out of the baking dish using the parchment paper overhang and cut into squares or bars.

14. Serve the lemon raspberry cheesecake bars chilled.

Chapter 7:

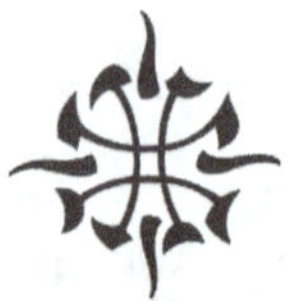

Incorporating exercise and physical activity:

Regular physical activity and exercise have numerous benefits for both physical and mental health. When it comes to cognitive function, exercise has been found to improve memory, attention, and overall brain health. It increases blood flow to the brain, promotes the growth of new neurons, and enhances the release of chemicals that support brain health and function.

To incorporate exercise into your routine, you can try activities such as brisk walking, jogging, cycling, swimming, dancing, or participating in sports. Aim for at least 150 minutes of moderate-intensity aerobic exercise or 75 minutes of vigorous-intensity exercise per week, along with strength training exercises at least twice a week. Find activities you enjoy and make them a regular part of your schedule.

Stress management techniques:

High levels of stress can negatively impact cognitive function and overall well-being. Implementing effective stress management techniques can help reduce stress and improve cognitive performance. Here are some techniques to consider:

- Practice relaxation techniques such as deep breathing exercises, meditation, or yoga.

- Engage in regular physical activity, as exercise can help reduce stress.

- Prioritize and organize tasks to avoid feeling overwhelmed.

- Set aside time for hobbies, interests, and activities you enjoy.

- Maintain a healthy work-life balance.

- Seek support from friends, family, or a mental health professional if needed.

Adequate sleep is crucial for optimal cognitive function. During sleep, the brain consolidates memories, processes information, and rejuvenates itself. Lack of sleep or poor-quality sleep can impair attention, concentration, memory, and decision-making abilities. To improve sleep quality:

- Establish a consistent sleep schedule, going to bed and waking up at the same time each day.

- Create a sleep-friendly environment that is dark, quiet, and comfortable.

- Limit exposure to electronic devices, especially before bedtime.

- Avoid consuming caffeine and large meals close to bedtime.

- Practice relaxation techniques to help you unwind before sleep.

Engaging in mental stimulation and challenging activities can help keep your brain sharp and improve cognitive function. Here are some suggestions:

- Solve puzzles and crosswords.

- Play strategy games such as chess or Sudoku.

- Learn a new skill or hobby, such as playing a musical instrument or painting.

- Read books, engage in meaningful discussions, or join a book club.

- Engage in social activities that require mental engagement, such as group discussions or debates.

Remember, maintaining a healthy lifestyle that includes regular exercise, stress management, quality sleep, and mental stimulation can contribute to improved cognitive function and overall well-being.

Chapter 8

Embracing the Menopause Brain Journey:

Menopause is a natural phase in a woman's life that brings about hormonal changes and can have an impact on various aspects of health, including cognitive function. Many women experience changes in memory, attention, and concentration during menopause, often referred to as "menopause brain" or "brain fog." It's important to understand that these changes are temporary and part of the natural transition. Here are some tips for embracing the menopause brain journey:

1. Educate yourself: Learn about the cognitive changes that can occur during menopause. Understanding that these changes are normal can help you approach them with a positive mindset and reduce anxiety.

2. Stay mentally active: Engage in activities that stimulate your brain. Read books, solve puzzles, play brain games, or learn something new. Keeping your mind active can help maintain cognitive function and promote brain health.

3. Manage stress: Menopause can be accompanied by increased stress levels, which can affect cognitive function. Find effective stress management techniques that work for you, such as deep breathing exercises, meditation, or engaging in activities you enjoy.

4. Prioritize sleep: Sleep disturbances are common during menopause and can impact cognitive function. Establish a regular sleep routine and create a sleep-friendly environment to improve the quality of your sleep. If

necessary, consult with a healthcare professional for guidance on managing sleep issues.

5. Practice self-care: Take care of your overall well-being. Eat a balanced diet, engage in regular physical activity, and prioritize self-care activities that promote relaxation and reduce stress.

6. Seek support: Connect with other women going through similar experiences. Join support groups or online communities where you can share your journey, ask questions, and receive support from others who understand what you're going through.

7. Talk to your healthcare provider: If you're concerned about your cognitive function or experiencing significant difficulties, discuss your symptoms with your healthcare provider. They can provide guidance, address any underlying health concerns, and offer strategies or treatments that may help.

Remember, menopause is a unique journey for every woman, and embracing the changes, including those related to cognitive function, can help you navigate this phase with greater ease and acceptance.

www.ingramcontent.com/pod-product-compliance
Lightning Source LLC
Chambersburg PA
CBHW072246260726
48659CB00004BA/1374